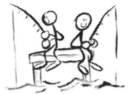

**This Ice Cream is Delicious**

**A Guide for Alzheimer's**

Second Edition

Published by

Atlanta Let's Go L.L.C.

© Copyright May 2015

by Henry F. Watts Jr.

ISBN: 978-0-9906063-0-7

Manufactured in the United States of America

# This Ice Cream is Delicious

## A Guide for Alzheimer's

Henry F. Watts Jr.

Let's Go

Atlanta Georgia

This book is dedicated to those who have cared for or are caring for someone who has Alzheimer's.

# Note to Reader

This book is written for anyone who is facing the challenge of caring for a loved one with dementia. I am intimately familiar with your struggle. My mother lived with Alzheimer's for eight years until she died in October 2008. When she was diagnosed, I was 32 and I didn't have a clue what to do or where to go. I didn't know how to get or even ask for help. I worried all the time and I had serious doubts about my ability to be a care-giver.

During those eight years, I learned the hard way about the difficulties of care-giving for someone with Alzheimer's. To honor my mother I started a company called Let's Go. I use what I learned to help families who are struggling with this devastating disease. I have now worked with over twenty families, and have cultivated relationships with the Alzheimer's Association and countless doctors, counselors, adult day care facilities and assisted living communities.

## What is Alzheimer's?

Alzheimer's is an irreversible brain disease that causes actual physical changes in the brain. There is no cure. As the disease progresses these physical changes can cause symptoms such as: Confusion, depression or withdrawal, irritability, aggression, mood swings, short and long term memory loss, trouble with speech, and loss of self-confidence.

Since we all think, act and react differently for a 1000 different reasons, these symptoms can vary from patient to patient.

Because the complexities are so difficult for *everyone* to understand, I don't spend too much time trying to answer "un-answerable" questions. Right out of the gate we'll start with suggestions, recommendations and ways to cope and live through this complicated disease. This book does cover the different stages of Alzheimer's but with a heavy emphasis on the early ones; the stages where the choices you make really can affect the quality of life for both you and the person you are caring for.

## Alzheimer's – A Family Disease

Alzheimer's is a disease that can put a heavy burden on care-givers. It is also a disease that can take hold of a family and relentlessly sabotage everyone's life.

*I'm hoping this book will allow everyone to see what each of you is going through, from understanding what the primary care-giver is coping with, right down to the effects on the grandkids. I wrote this book to help family and friends, from the youngest to the "young at heart", to care and cope for themselves and their loved one, stay united and not just react to this disease.*

## The Day Your Loved One is Diagnosed, What Do You Do?

Important decisions made in the immediate aftermath of a diagnosis – when your family is grieving – can help keep your loved one active and engaged. Stories about what I experienced as a care-giver for my mother, interviews with experts, and anecdotes about the families I have worked with, will hopefully offer you some practical advice, as well as words of support and understanding in your struggle.

My goal is to help you know what to expect and to guide you along the way, so that your path might be less frightening than the one I found myself on fourteen years ago.

Alzheimer's is very, very difficult. I sincerely hope this book can make a difference in your life.

Henry F. Watts Jr.
May 2015
Atlanta, GA

# CONTENTS

# Reading Help

- I hope this book will be helpful to all care-givers, especially those who are caring for someone who is in the early to moderate stages of Alzheimer's disease (AD). Based on my experience, I find that the information about the early to moderate stages is the most neglected and overlooked.

- I have changed most of my clients' names as I want to respect their privacy.

- I have tried to write the book as chronologically as possible from early-stage AD to the end. Categorizing AD is difficult because everyone is different. The early and late stages are more predictable, but everything in between is not.

- Throughout the book I have used phone conversations, emails, and texts from my clients' spouses or family members and friends. By including these, I hope to give you a broader perspective (not only my experience but theirs as well).

- This book contains what I know about AD and how it affects families. You won't find many scientific explanations in here about AD.

- Even though Alzheimer's is a very specific form of dementia, it is responsible for more than fifty percent of the cases of dementia. **I have worked with people that have been diagnosed with Frontotemporal Dementia (FTD), Mixed Dementia, Lewy Body Dementia, and have recently starting working with someone who has Parkinson's Disease Dementia (PDD).** A number of people I have worked with had initially been diagnosed with Alzheimer's, but as the disease progressed the diagnosis also changed. I think a lot of information in the book is relevant and appropriate for Alzheimer's as well as other types of irreversible dementia.

- There is theory and then there is your real world. I want you to know that if I have said something that seems "ridiculous" to you, my apologies. Although it might not pertain to you or your loved one, it may be just the ticket for someone else since everyone who has AD is affected differently.

- I recommend keeping an open mind. Don't be afraid to try new things throughout your experience with Alzheimer's.

# Abbreviations

The following are terms that you will find throughout the book.

**AD**: Alzheimer's disease.

**YLO**: Your Loved One. There is not a word in the English language that explains "the person with dementia that you love and are caring for." Until that word is defined, "YLO" is what I'll use.

**Caregiver**: Usually the family member who is primarily caring for YLO. This could also mean a paid care-giver. You will know.

**The Lowman**: The Lowman Home in White Rock, South Carolina, is the assisted living facility where my mother lived for three years.

**Home: Assisted Living Facility**: Thirty years ago they were all called "homes." Now there are numerous types of facilities but generally I will still refer to them as a "Home."

**Clients**: The people I work with. I don't like this term, but I have not found any other word I can use that best suits. They are not my patients; I'm not a doctor. Throughout this book I will interchange the terms friends, pals, and clients. I call them my friends all the time because they are. You will know who I am talking about.

**Me**: "The Caregiver." I was a care-giver for my mom. Now, I'm not really a "care-giver," because I don't give care. I am more of a companion. For the sake of keeping things simple, I'll call myself a "care-giver."

# Introduction

Before Mom was diagnosed, I was living a terrific life. Great parents, the best friends a guy could have. I traveled. I played in a few bands. I had a great "slacker" job with absolutely no stress. I was 32 and didn't have a care in the world... I was caught like a deer in headlights.

Alzheimer's crashed into me like a Buick.

I know all about that lonely feeling. The one where you think you are the only one in the world – and you constantly say to yourself, "How in the world am I going to get through this?"

Some of the content in this book might seem obvious to you, but none of it was obvious to me when my mom was first diagnosed. I didn't have a clue what I was doing. There was no "guide." I was just doing the best I could and I stumbled through a lot of it. You might have a handle on AD. As you read a few things in here, you might even roll your eyes a bit and think, "How did someone miss this?" I overlooked and missed some of the simplest tasks because I was in a state of perpetual worry. The pressure is staggering and it's certainly enough to warp your thinking. You might have it "together" and you might understand what you are up against, but I bet most of you are just like I was – OVERWHELMED.

I have worked exclusively with people who have dementia for eight years now. I have a close relationship with the Atlanta Alzheimer's Association, have been to over ten adult day care centers in Atlanta, probably twenty assisted living homes and ten memory care facilities – with friends in all of them. I placed my mom into an assisted living facility, and when it was time have helped other families do the same.

I spend many hours a week with families struggling with AD, helping them navigate the tremendous responsibility of care-giving for someone who has Alzheimer's. Invitations into the life of the family have helped to develop strategies that get their loved one out of the house and back in the action. We pursue their interests and look for adventure. When you add all of this to my experience with my mom, I know my way around the world of Alzheimer's as well as any, and better than most.

There is no standard journey for anyone who has AD. There are some general similarities along the way, but everyone will be affected differently, and every family has its own unique situation and response to this challenge.

For the eight years after my mother was diagnosed I had a difficult time focusing on the disease. The challenge was so foreign to me. One minute I would understand what we were up against and then the next, I wouldn't know what to do or how to help her. The progression of this disease can be subtle but at the same time it can be overwhelming. After working with so many families I know that most people feel this way...

Everyone feels lost.

The most difficult thing for every new care-giver to understand – I know it was for me – is that: Alzheimer's is an irreversible brain disease. It's not like cancer, where you go to a doctor and then follow a linear path to get better. Because there is no cure and the disease is so complex it has a way of creating an indescribable confusion for the care-giver, the family and friends.

## What Do You Do?

Writing this book has allowed me to focus on the root of the problems that Alzheimer's can cause a family and now I know; there is a path... and you need a good map. This Ice Cream is Delicious is a map; one I wish had been there for me.

A clear vision of the road ahead will allow you to cut through some of the "static." Understanding the possibilities and realizing the limitations that might come with each stage will allow you to focus on care-giving. This book will allow you collect your own thoughts, help you develop your own strategies for coping and you might, just might, be able to avoid some of the anxiety and exhaustion that causes so much of the sadness this disease can bring.

The most important goal of this book is to prepare and guide you through the details and difficult decisions you will face, so that you can concentrate on what matters most: **Enjoying the time you have with your loved one.**

---

I was visiting my mom one spring afternoon. Together we were doing yard work, raking leaves and planting tomatoes. We were having a great day doing what we had always done together every spring. After a while, Mom walked into the house and closed the front door. I heard it lock. She then closed the side door. I wasn't quite sure what to make of this so I knocked on the front door. When she opened it, she said, "Well, hey Henry! It's so great to see you... come on in!"

That was the moment I knew.

By winter, my aunts Mary Beth and Evelyn and I took Mom to see a neurologist. We all knew something was wrong. Her memory was just not the same. She was diagnosed with dementia, probably Alzheimer's. I remember the phone call. I remember where I was, the time of day – and I remember the feeling.

In the pages before you is some information that I wish I had known on that day.

---

# Now

## 1.

There is no other feeling in the world when you find out someone you love has been diagnosed with Alzheimer's. The sadness is profound and life changing. I have heard many family members say that they would gladly trade places with the one who has Alzheimer's. To watch someone suffering for so long is devastating. Even the greatest writer wouldn't be able to capture that in words.

What I'll offer are "possibilities."

I want you to know there is help and there is hope. There are things you can do right now that will in some cases dramatically affect the happiness and quality of life for your loved one, you and your family.

### You – The Care-giver

The most difficult aspect of dementia for a care-giver is the helplessness you will probably feel by the lack of control over what is happening. I hope in these next two chapters to restore some confidence and offer a few ideas that might enable you to develop more control over the situation, **right now.**

So your loved one has been diagnosed with Alzheimer's... Just like you, I ignored the signs (everyone does), but now it's time to get this started.

One of the first steps you can take is to help YLO retain a good quality of life by building strength against the advancements of AD. By helping with nutrition, exercise, and socialization, you can give YLO a much better chance at defending against these advancements. Establishing and maintaining a healthy routine will keep YLO in shape physically and mentally. Eating nutritious food increases energy for exercise, which improves appetite and results in better sleep. Feeling good physically will allow more opportunities for getting out, socializing and staying active.

## Nutrition

Until there is a cure for Alzheimer's, the best we can do is take care of ourselves and pursue a healthful life. Proper nutrition is important for better brain function, overall health, and maintaining a healthy body to fight off the effects of AD.

### An Interview with a Dietician

Corinne, whom I have known since high school, is a registered and licensed dietitian with a Master's in Human Nutrition.

**Bio**: Corinne Cates, MS RD LD has over thirteen years of experience as a registered dietitian. **Corinne has extensive experience addressing the nutritional concerns of dementia patients in Geriatrics and long-term care settings.** She has served as the chief clinical dietitian and director of nutrition in facilities that specialize in treating patients with dementia.

Hello Corinne,

I have a few questions about healthy eating and its importance in overall health, particularly as it pertains to Alzheimer's patients.

> **Q. (Henry) If you knew someone who had just been diagnosed with Alzheimer's, would you make recommendations to their diet? What would they be?**

> A. *(Corinne) Yes I would – definitely. I know that current research indicates that a Mediterranean diet reduces the risk of Alzheimer's, so certainly incorporating those eating habits would be beneficial.*

> *The Mediterranean diet emphasizes several important habits: Eating primarily plant-based foods, such as fruits and vegetables, whole grains, legumes and nuts. Eating plenty of fresh produce (vegetables and whole fruits) in an array of colors across the spectrum provides a host of phytochemicals (antioxidants, vitamins, and minerals) crucial to maintaining brain and cardiovascular health. The colors found in fruits and vegetables indicate foods rich in a variety of antioxidants and vital vitamins and minerals. Eating dark green leafy vegetables (such as vegetables from the brassica family like cauliflower, broccoli, and Brussels sprouts) and deep, rich-colored berries like blueberries and blackberries each day maximizes nutritional protection. Decreasing the consumption of meat and full fat dairy products is beneficial for the cardiovascular system and*

*brain health since it decreases the amount of saturated fats in our diet.*

*The cornerstone of this diet is: eating fish and poultry twice a week, saturated fatty acids from oils such as olive oil and canola oil instead of butter (saturated fats) or margarine (trans fats), omega-3 fatty acids (from cold water fish such as salmon, tuna, mackerel, and herring), and vegetable sources (such as green leafy vegetables, flaxseed oil, and nuts (walnuts). These types of fats are important for proper brain growth and development. They make up a large part of cell membranes, which serve to protect cells from damage. They also reduce inflammation.*

**Q.** **If someone with AD were to lose his or her appetite, are there things that can be done to restore appetite?**

*A.* *Loss of appetite and weight loss are symptoms of the disease process. Assisting your loved one to consume good, wholesome foods would be preferable, but not always possible. Someone with Alzheimer's may refuse foods that they have always loved and eaten or, at times, refuse to eat at all. In this case, any foods or beverages they are willing to consume would be the best bet. For instance, if your loved one wants to eat mostly ice cream, you could try making a milkshake and adding fresh fruit and protein powder for extra nutrition. You can also make a smoothie or milkshake using a supplement such as Ensure of Glucerna (if diabetic). In the instance of a low appetite and/ or weight loss, the emphasis switches to simply getting nutrients in the individual in the manner they will accept it.*

**Q.** **The brain is much more capable of growth and repair than we once thought. How does proper nutrition play a part in the brain actually being able to repair itself?**

*A.* *Glial cells are non-neuronal cells that provide physical and nutritional support to neurons. Their name is derived from the Greek word for "glue". There are roughly 10 to 50 times as many glial cells in the brain as neurons. These cells transport nutrients to neurons and provide myelin (protective covering) to neurons in the central nervous system. The proper fats including essential fatty acids such as Omega-3s are crucial to supporting their functioning. Current research is discovering more about the role of glial cells in the brain, including the role and importance of the chemical signals they use for communication to neurons. Glial cells are thought to regulate the flow of information through the brain. Consuming plenty of unsaturated fats, from vegetable sources, while avoiding saturated fats mostly from animal sources is the key to promoting proper lipid (Lipid) functioning.*

*I think it is sufficient to say that the brain has regenerative capabilities that were never conceived of in the past. This is an even greater incentive to eat a diet filled with "good, healthy" fats and devoid of "processed, convenience foods."*

**Thanks Corinne! This is great information. I couldn't help but notice all the foods you have suggested are *real* foods.**

## Serve It!

Make the most of the healthy foods you know YLO likes. If she likes cole slaw, use the best slaw ingredients. Instead of white potatoes, try sweet potatoes, which are one of the most nutritious foods out there. On occasion, try brown rice instead of white. At a restaurant get the big salad, not just the side salad. Do your best to avoid fried foods – choose the baked chicken instead. Slowly introduce more fruits and vegetables. Be sure to keep YLO well-hydrated with lots of water, and limit the soft drinks (if you can). Try and replace any sugary drinks with fresh, 100% fruit juice (watch out for juices that are mostly high fructose corn syrup). Serve fresh foods whenever possible, especially fresh fish for healthy Omega-3s. Cut out fatty meat and watch the processed food. Do everything you can to help YLO eat well and feel good.

## Smoothies

Everyone has a blender. Most everyone likes milkshakes. Make a healthy milkshake without the "milkshake" and start a regimen with a smoothie in the morning. If there is some resistance use a non-see-through cup with a lid and a straw. Start simple: apple, banana, maybe a little peanut butter for protein. Use fruit juice, milk, rice or almond milk. If it doesn't catch on, just say the doctor recommends one every morning. Tell them that it will help improve their memory, which in a way, is true. Drinking a smoothie could make a lot of difference in YLO's mood and energy level. When you start getting a good routine down, try new things. Carrots and apples are a great combo and berries contain all the good omegas and antioxidants. Even spinach and kale work well with the right combination, and can't be detected. Dark chocolate (at least 80% cocoa) is great for energy, eases inflammation and promotes heart health. Protein powder is a great addition for people who aren't getting enough protein.

## Vitamins and Supplements

I usually recommend a few vitamins and supplements to my clients because a regimen could help supply their body with what they might miss nutritionally. Vitamin D, E, B12, B6 and Omega 3's. Everyone's physical make-up is different, so before you take anything, consult with your doctor.

## Vitamin D

In a small pilot study, a team of US researchers has discovered how vitamin D3, a form of vitamin D, and Omega 3 fatty acids may help the immune system clear the brain of amyloid plaques, one of the physical hallmarks of Alzheimer's disease.[1]

## Vitamin E

Vitamin E is an antioxidant, protecting the body from oxidative damage that can accelerate aging. The Linus Pauling Institute (Oregon State University, Micronutrient Research for Optimum Health) states that the brain is particularly subject to oxidative stresses, leading to conditions such as dementia and Alzheimer's disease. The institute reports that vitamin E levels have been found to be low in patients diagnosed with AD, and supplementing with 2,000 IU per day of vitamin E for two years slows the onset and progression of Alzheimer's. Vitamin E is also available in food sources such as nuts, seeds, boiled spinach, and broccoli.[2]

## B Vitamins

The blood work for the Alzheimer's patient shows high levels of homocysteine, an amino acid in the blood. Researchers at Oxford University report that high levels of this amino acid are a risk factor for conditions such as brain atrophy and impairment of brain function, including AD. The Oxford study, published in the September 8, 2010, issue of PLoS One, also states that treatment with B vitamins, particularly folic acid, B12, and B6, slows the rate at which brain function declines by lowering homocysteine levels. This action of B vitamins may also slow the onset of AD.[2]

## Omega 3's

Research has also linked high intake of omega-3s to a possible reduction in risk of dementia or cognitive decline. The chief omega-3 in the brain is DHA, which is found in the fatty membranes that surround nerve cells, especially at the microscopic junctions where cells connect to one another. Theories about why omega-3s might influence dementia risk include their benefit for the heart and blood vessels; anti-inflammatory effects; and support and protection of nerve cell membranes.[3]

## Water

Dehydration takes a toll on everyone fighting an illness, but when someone has AD, being dehydrated can really affect their mental health. I have seen a client becoming dehydrated due to pneumonia change into an unrecognizable mental state only to be brought back by a visit to the ER and an IV. Drinking plenty of water is key to optimum health.

## Difficulties in Eating Healthy

Introducing new food and breaking lifelong habits are very difficult, especially when AD is involved. There are a million books written about proper nutrition and supplements and obviously these diets work great for those who are open minded about eating. Some of the people I have worked with have consciously changed their diet in order to try and get better, so I do have clients who eat healthy. However, some of them eat BBQ and French fries, and drink Coca-Cola. And, if they couldn't, they would rather starve.

Cutting back on processed food and staying out of the middle aisles in a grocery store would be preferable, but getting some people with AD to eat healthy can be an unsolvable mystery. If you have tried to get YLO to eat healthier and it's just not working, **it's not your fault**. When I take my clients out to the barbecue and burger joints in Atlanta, I am impressed with how many sophisticated and healthy options they offer, but that doesn't mean my guys will eat them.

Do what you can to change YLO's diet over time but if there is a lot of resistance to new and healthy food then, as Corinne told us, stick with what you know and realize that at least he or she is eating and getting some nutrition. The food they have eaten has kept them going this long! Maybe it's possible to make some small changes. That is why I asked Corinne to recommend some impact foods that could play a role in possibly improving diet and eating healthier.

## Exercise

Patients with early Alzheimer's disease who exercise regularly saw less deterioration in the areas of the brain which control memory, according to a study released at the 2008 International Conference on Alzheimer's Disease in Chicago.[4]

Exercise and physical fitness have been shown to slow down age-related brain-cell death for healthy older adults too. Exercise may help slow brain shrinkage in people with early Alzheimer's disease.[4]

For most of their life, YLO probably got up every day and went to work. With the advancing AD, they probably get up and find that there isn't much to do except watch TV, especially if no one else is home. YLO needs to burn some energy somehow or they are going to be restless. If they get a chance to exercise, they will eat and sleep better. Sleep is a time when the brain restores itself (brain plasticity). Without good sleep, they might be edgy and depression might advance. Not exercising could lead to a decreased appetite. No appetite means no intake of the nutrients YLO needs to fight AD. **It's all a cycle**.

Setting up times to exercise together is a great way to spend time with YLO. Get moving and keep moving: Walking, swimming, tennis, using an exercise bike, martial arts (disciplines like Tai Chi are exceptional for focus and concentration), stretching, treadmill, golf, and yard work. All are great forms of exercise.

Walking is #1. **A routine of walking is the most important thing you can establish.** Studies have shown that walking five miles a week can help preserve grey matter in the brain. Find a gym or a facility that is indoors where you can walk if it's too hot or cold. I walk with Edward all the time, and he loves to walk anywhere, especially the Atlanta Botanical Garden. We take hikes up Kennesaw Mountain and at state and city parks. Name it and we have been there to walk and are probably on the way to one right now. Start making walks part of YLO's routine as soon as you can.

I play tennis with Tom every Tuesday. He hadn't played in ten years but he was a good player as a young man. He played tournaments and in an Atlanta tennis league (ALTA). I had no idea if he could still hit the ball, but we took the chance that he might and soon found out he could! I was relieved. He has trouble remembering anyone's name except his wife's and struggles to finish his sentences, but when that racket is in his hand, he is king. He is in control. He loves it! He can barely converse but he can hit that tennis ball. Since we discovered tennis, when we get off the court I can tell he feels great. His confidence is back. He talks the whole way home.

I take a few of my guys out to the golf range. At first they are a little disappointed in their play, but they still enjoy being there, especially if the weather is nice. The more we go, the more they appreciate being there. I am amazed at the success some of my clients have in hitting the ball just by introducing shorter clubs. Most of the time they forget about what they used to be able to do and concentrate on what they can do now. I always tell them they hit the ball a lot better than the last time and emphasize that their swing looks good. When they drive a good ball, I can see the satisfaction on their faces.

**Not getting any exercise can bring on multiple problems:** Unused energy could find a different outlet – agitated or aggressive behavior (especially in men). Another is loss of balance. Important muscle groups that support us go unused – that can bring on falls.

Exercise can affect almost every aspect of mood, confidence and energy level. I hear this sort of thing from my clients' families all the time: "Robin was so much more relaxed when we got home after our walk." Exercise and physical activity increase oxygen intake, get the blood flowing and helps the brain with angiogenesis, the creation of new blood vessels. Another guide you can use is, "What is good for the heart is good for the brain."

**It's been proven countless times that exercising every day lowers anxiety and improves mental outlook – key in the fight against AD.**

But, how is a 68-year-old man going to all of a sudden go to the gym and like it? I started working with a guy whose family thought that exercise, the social interaction with the trainer, and the health food at the gym would help him. His family complained to me that he didn't ever want to go to the gym. They thought he was just being difficult. They had made all these great arrangements for him to get into shape and he wasn't cooperating.

I bet this is what he was thinking: "All of a sudden I am in the gym. I never used to go to any gym! Who is this guy who is telling me to do these complicated exercises? We stay here forever. The food is bad and I don't want to do this anymore. I'm not interested. I'd rather stay at home where my wife needs me."

The best way to get an activity accomplished and made enjoyable is look at YLO's life and what they enjoyed and then apply those elements. Think it through. Sit down for an hour and write down everything he or she enjoyed doing. Maybe out of that list, there will be a good idea of what they might enjoy doing now.

Because the nature of the disease, we all scramble for activities and exercises for our loved ones, especially those who might have become disinterested in things they have always enjoyed. I have found the best way to introduce or reintroduce someone with AD to exercise is to take it slow and consider this:

The overall experience is more important than the specific activity.

    a.   A walk or bike ride in the morning when it's 75 degrees, maybe lunch after at a favorite (low key) restaurant.

    b.   A walk or bike ride at noon when it's 110... after doing six errands.

If I want more experiences for my clients, then I have to make sure the conditions are right for the whole outing. I look at it this way: The entire outing is ONE experience. Also, **too many activities lasting too long is counterproductive.** Don't feel as though you are responsible for a full day's worth of activities. If you can get one to three meaningful hours in a day for someone who has become disinterested in most everything, it's a win all around. If you are successful and they are engaged in something for even just one hour – that's terrific! Next month go for two!

## An Interview with Tonja

Finding someone to interview who was a fitness instructor for people who have early memory loss was difficult. Most senior centers offer exercise classes, but the participants must be mentally able to participate without any disruption. I think that's why, in general, finding things to do for someone with AD can be difficult. I have met several people who work with those with advanced stages of AD but I was looking for someone whose primary clients have early-to-moderate AD and can still exercise but might need close supervision. After an extensive search, I found Tonja. She offers classes that specifically include people with AD and she has some great ideas about getting people up and moving.

**Bio**: Tonja Cash is a certified wellness coach, group fitness instructor, and personal trainer who develops fitness programs for dementia sufferers (www.fundamentallyfit.com). Tonja was highly recommended by the Dekalb County Senior Center – Senior Connections. She told me this when we met:

> "I have a personal passion for working with Alzheimer's patients and their families because of family history. Many times I wished someone had HONESTLY explained to me and my family the physical, emotional, financial and spiritual components of this disease."

Hello Tonja,

Thank you so much for participating in this interview.

**Q. (Henry) Are there exercise classes for people with early-to-moderate stage dementia?**

A. *(Tonja) Yes, but first I suggest that anyone starting a new exercise plan should have medical clearance. Those with dementia will have the same physical fitness – cardiovascular, strength and flexibility objectives as others in their age group. The problem I see is that most physical fitness programs are totally self-propelled or large group experiences. A self-propelled program means the exerciser does an exercise program without assistance, by oneself. This is how most people exercise in a gym setting. A group exercise class is instructor led with all participants following specific instructions. Neither of these environments work well for those with dementia. They need either one-on-one training or a very small group exercise experience with someone who understands not only their physical, but their cognitive abilities. What I offer in my class is: Strength training – free weights, bands, body weight, circuit weight equipment; Cardiovascular training – walking, stationary bicycle, elliptical, dance; Flexibility – yoga and stretching.*

*If they have a care-giver, I would suggest water aerobics. There are a number of reasons why.*

*First of all it's good for all activity levels. This is important because as people age, there are usually physical impairments. Water aerobics is very easy on the joints and great for those with balance issues. This allows people to continue a familiar exercise activity even when they are facing declining health. There is sometimes a strong social* component in many classes, along with a feeling of physical freedom and independence in the water. There are also defined boundaries of the pool which means that there is little risk of someone wandering off and, for many institutional deep water pools, a life guard is present.

**Q.** **Some of the men and women I work with have never been to a gym and have never exercised in the traditional sense. Like me, they even have a hard time saying the word "yoga." I am always looking for ways to get them to exercise which helps to build up their appetites and in turn sleep better. What are your suggestions about how to get them involved in an exercise program?**

A. *I would say incorporate familiar activities. I think the care-giver needs to be aware that the usual exercise motivational factors – looking good (ego), losing/maintaining weight (health/ego), and sleep concerns (health) – usually are not going to work for someone with memory or brain disease issues. I think it's a comprehension issue. I try to meet people where they are and not where I want them to be. I do functional fitness, which means I ask people to do things that make sense to them. For example, most people are familiar with sports such as tennis, bowling and softball. Sometimes the activities have to be modified while keeping the fitness goals intact. Playing basketball on a court may be changed to throwing objects into baskets. These activities use shoulder range-of-motion exercises (reaching up and down) without me calling it exercise. A bicycle ride in a calm setting may be done on a stationary bike with background music or TV.*

*The goal is to mimic the physical activities needed to remain independent. With the patient, I also focus on strengthening the core muscles. Again, I highly recommend balance exercises in the water. Walking is one of the low impact exercises available. Walking with a dog can be good exercise and fun. It also gives those with dementia a sense of purpose. You can even borrow pets to walk. Un-crowded malls can also be a fun safe place to walk.*

Q. **I know you have had success in getting people to exercise who normally wouldn't be interested and this can be difficult especially since as you have said ego might not play a role in them participating. What is your main strategy in your program?**

A. *My primary goal is to help those diagnosed with dementia remain physically active as long as possible. I provide individual and small group activities that address the physical, cognitive, and socialization needs of those with AD and their care-givers. My strategy is to provide a variety of activity options that can be utilized throughout all stages of dementia. These adaptive exercise programs provide continuity and can be started in the early, moderate, or later stages of dementia.*

Q. **What are some of your favorite resources?**

A. *I would say any governmental (ex. nihseniorhealth.gov) and medical review websites would be good. I prefer the National Institute of Health/ CDC type publications because the information is medically reviewed **and not just public relations stories planted by drug or healthcare related companies.** Some hospitals (Mayo Clinic) and universities have good information. I think with a medically fragile population it's important to use resources that are carefully sourced and researched. In fact, a lot of for-profit (and non-profit) entities use the federal government guidelines/research in their publications. I would rather go directly to the source.*

These answers are great Tonja. As I was reading them you uncovered a few things I really had never thought about before, especially the motivational factors – health/ego. I really appreciate your hard work and what you do for the community.

**One Last Note About Exercise**

There comes a time when legs and arms don't quite work as well as they used to. I have had a few wives insist that I reintroduce golf to their husbands, but I knew that wasn't going to work. YLO needs to be mentally and physically capable for the activity. If you think he or she is capable and would have fun, give it a shot. I have taken guys out to the golf driving range to within two months of their last day on Earth. Some people keep that balance and eye/hand coordination intact. It depends on the person, the disease, and what part of the brain the disease is attacking.

## Socialization

Along with good nutrition and proper exercise, making sure YLO stays active and social is crucial. A lot of people with AD start to withdraw. I completely understand. I would withdraw too if I wasn't so sure about what I could or couldn't do anymore. Their confidence is shaky and they are at an extremely high risk for depression. That is why finding the things that they enjoy and making sure they do them and stay active and social is so important.

With my experience helping people who have AD and their families, I've learned a lot about the strategy and creativity that goes into keeping YLO active and happy. I'll give you some suggestions for some basic ways to start establishing routine activities, but the most important thing to do is to remember YLO's individual interests, talents, and past experiences when you are working on ways to keep them busy.

My experience working with Scott was rewarding, because it was so clear that my efforts to keep him active were making a difference. We became great friends and did all kinds of activities together; we went to air shows, car shows, bowling, guy movies, the driving range etc. I even helped his family out during his daughter's wedding. Seeing him walk his daughter down the aisle... not a dry eye in the room.

Marie is a devout Catholic. Her church is very important to her. Before I began working with her, she had been going to church sporadically even though it meant so much to her. I help Marie get to the church she has been attending for over sixty years – where she was married and where her children were baptized. Marie remembers all the hymns and always sees a friend at Mass. It is a huge victory for her to stand up and take communion every week, just as she has done all her life. We get dressed up before and have lunch after. Some weeks we go two and three times. Our church routine has become the highlight of her week, and I have been able to earn Marie's trust by helping her to stay active in something that means so much to her.

Ellen comes from a huge family of artists in New York, so I thought she would enjoy cultural events. On our first outing, I decided to take her to the Carlos Theater at Emory University for a classical music performance. I wasn't sure how it would go. The program was divided into two parts. The first was a beautiful, upbeat waltz. My favorite. Fun music. The second part was a challenging, dark, and intense piece, and I thought, "Uh-oh. Is Ellen enjoying this?" When it was over, she said, "What a wonderful show! The second part was my favorite! Let's come back tomorrow night!" I felt great that I had been able to draw her out with an activity that suited her.

## Eating Out

The best visits I have with my clients involve one or two planned activities and a great meal out. Going out to lunch and dinner is very important to us but if YLO is becoming less interested in eating out or you are becoming less interested in eating out with them(!), then here are a few suggestions that have worked for me.

- Find that great waitress/waiter who can make everyone comfortable. They will know the food YLO likes, so ordering won't be confusing. If the staff knows what's going on, servers can be prepared to make some effort to communicate if things get frustrating.

- Scout out a location. I have walked into restaurants and said "My pal and I will be having lunch here. He has dementia and he might say a few things you might not understand. Can I pick out a spot and let the server know what is going on?" It's always a great experience when the service is on board with all the humorous moments and "interesting" comments. I have a few guys that always turn the dining experience into a riot. A fun one.

- Invite friends along whenever you can, so YLO stays connected to his or her social circle.

- Avoid anxiety by staying away from loud, crowded restaurants. They are confusing and pose too many distractions. I can't hear myself think in some of these places so imagine what YLO is going through.

- There is usually a more relaxed atmosphere at the bar in a restaurant. The TV's are on and the bar tenders are always friendly. Lunch or dinner, all my guys love to sit there.

- If possible eat early or eat late. Avoid the lunch rush. I recommend going around 11:30 or after 1:00pm.

- And, of course, talk about the good life. Stay away from topics that aren't friendly.

## Volunteering – A Sense of Purpose

Volunteering is a great way to spend time with someone who has early memory loss. If they can handle a simple task and carry on a short conversation, you are in business. Volunteering gets them out of the house, helps others who are less fortunate, and develops new friendships. The right volunteer work could be a real confidence booster.

My favorite volunteer activity is Meals On Wheels. At one time in the short history of Let's Go, I was doing Meals On Wheels with three guys – Tuesday, Wednesday, and Thursday. I drive but we each participate. If they can remember the route, they help navigate. We both hand out the meals and sometimes we're invited inside for a short chat with some of our recipients. We have developed some great relationships. Our pal Charlie is a recipient and we always look forward to seeing him. Tom and I always put him last on our route because we end up staying for an hour! We three have become good friends. On another route with one of my clients, we deliver to four Holocaust survivors; my client is Jewish so that carries an added meaning. They don't speak English and we don't speak Russian but somehow we all became friends.

My clients get to volunteer, they don't have to drive, I usually lead the conversation and direct where it's going. Because we always have to push off towards the next delivery, most of the conversations are short. We have also helped a few folks in building their ramps for wheelchair access and helped when I knew something wasn't quite right health-wise with some of our recipients. By being involved in Meals On Wheels, my clients are helping the community and they know it. It gives them structure and purpose, and they love it.

A good way to get a grandchild involved with his/her grandfather/ grandmother would be to ask him or her if they would be interested in making $40 by taking YLO to do Meals On Wheels once a week. YLO gets out of the house, you get three hours to yourself, and that grandkid gets to know his grandparent a little better while making a little cash and doing something worthwhile.

The local food bank is always looking for volunteers to help pack the bags. My mom and her friend Don volunteered at a food bank until she entered assisted living, and I know they enjoyed it. Again, spending time doing something worthwhile.

Visiting assisted living facilities is another great way to offer service and socialize. Short visits to residents lift their spirits and keep them company. First I stop by and ask the staff if there is a resident who might appreciate a visit (maybe one who might not receive many visitors). I then ask this resident if it would be OK to bring my friend by who has AD but would enjoy meeting and visiting with them. When we go, my clients know they are helping someone and they feel involved. This isn't for everyone, but I work with a few guys that love to talk and meet new people.

Everyone wins.

If you think he or she would like to be a volunteer, do not wait to get them involved. Volunteer programs almost always have an orientation class, which means paying attention for maybe an hour or more and possibly writing something. I recommend taking the orientation NOW, so you will have your badge and papers already done and he or she will be ready to start. I remember I worked with a real dog lover and I thought the dog-walking program at the Humane Society would be perfect. My wife used to volunteer there. It was a program where you take a dog out in the play area and play fetch and run around for a half hour with each dog. How perfect is that if you love dogs? So I called and found out that the orientation class is three hours long. It covers all the volunteering posts. No exceptions. My client couldn't possibly make it through that, but I bet a year ago he
could have.

## Dogs: Everyone's Best Friend

The people I work with love their dogs. I have seen a bond between my clients and their dog so strong you could write another book about it. Their dogs are the one and only one they can count on *all the time*. Dogs don't take the car keys away. Dogs don't make anyone go to the doctor. Dogs don't say things that are confusing. Dogs listen and they speak a language everyone knows and can understand. When you walk in the front door, a dog will treat you like you are a rock star, every time.

Why a dog? "Hey Allan, It's time for you to walk the dog." – Exercise. Walking a dog gets you out of the house to the see neighbors "Hey Allan! How's it going?" – Socialization. Dogs need someone to feed and take care of them – Responsibility. Dogs offer wonderful companionship and they are loyal and protective, which is perfect for someone struggling with AD.

> I'm sure the bonds are just as strong between our cat lovers, so no offense to our feline friends... but you can't walk a cat.

If you are dealing with early stage dementia and you think YLO would really appreciate a loyal companion, then go on down to the local Humane Society and pick out a two-year-old, housebroken, sweet, 40lb rescue and watch YLO change right before your eyes. Get an easy-going one that you know will be a great friend. Having a dog is a real commitment though, so don't take this decision lightly.

**Let's Go**

I work with families by assisting their loved ones in the continuation of an active life style. The name of my company says it all... Let's Go. My company's slogan: **Let us help make every minute count.** Finding activities to do with YLO in your town can be difficult but making the effort might make a huge difference in YLO's happiness and yours.

Make a list of everything in your area that you think YLO might enjoy so you have something to glance at when it's time to get out. Invite a friend to come along. Check your local university or college, churches and senior centers for programs.

**Places of interest:**

History, science, or art museums

The zoo

Botanical gardens

Art galleries

*Become members, you will go more.*

**Suggested walks:**

In the neighborhood

State park

City parks

By the river

Downtown

Local shopping mall

**Things of a particular interest:**

- High school band rehearsal.
- Dance classes – attend or watch.
- Fishing.
- Activities with fellow Veterans. Programs at a VFW post.
- Music: Live music programs in churches, music halls/venues.
- Theater: Plays or musicals in any number of theaters.
- Religious functions: Bible study, synagogue, J.C.C.
- Taking pictures: Grab a camera, head out for the day taking pictures.
- Painting: Take a class at one of the many studios around town.
- Garden Club: Attend flower shows.
- Dogs: Take a dog for a walk. Visit The Humane Society and play/walk/run one of their dogs.

**Physical fitness/sports:**

- Tennis. Watch or play.
- Golf: Driving range and hit a few. Attending golf tournaments. Miniature golf.
- Swimming.
- YMCA: Light stretching class.
- Sporting events/practice: High school, collage or professional. Football, baseball, basketball, tennis, soccer.

**Miscellaneous:**

- Darts, shoot a game of pool.
- Conventions: Record, Book, Watch, Antique, Car shows, etc.
- I have a friend whose step father has AD and they spend a lot of time in record stores flipping through records.
- Electronic, hardware, fish and tackle, and hobby stores. Some of my guys like to wander around all the guy stuff.
- Movies: We have an overpriced science museum that has an IMAX theater. Take a forty minute trip to the North Pole, a safari in Africa, outer space or under the sea. All of my clients love going.
- Walks: There is a unique trail by the Atlanta History Center with water falls and indigenous plants, five minutes from downtown Atlanta.
- I had a neighbor whose profession was playing piano during ballet rehearsals. I used to take my client Jill, who enjoyed the ballet, to rehearsals. It was perfect! She loved it.
- Museums: I have taken my clients to almost every museum large or small in a fifty mile radius. Railway Museum in Duluth, Delta Museum, etc. We have ended up at "museums" that are so small, you are lucky if they are open.

**Outside**

I usually have one or two clients who live in assisted living. I actually help families with the transition. Once they move in, I try to get my client involved with everything the facility has to offer including the "outings" they have.

These places are always looking for volunteers, especially for guy "stuff", so sometimes we take them to Braves baseball games, bowling, and I have even taken a few guys fishing. One thing I have noticed when we are out and it's raining, somehow, it's always fun. Might sound bizarre, but these people live in such a temperature controlled world that sometimes when they get out and get wet, it can be a real laugh.

One time at a particular memory care facility, we had ten people in a van, three people were in wheel chairs. There was a tremendous downpour and everyone got soaked going from the van to the restaurant, but when we all sat down everyone was in such a great mood. All smiling and happy, talking and swapping stories. Everyone seemed to be very aware. It was almost like being awakened from a sleep.

We get sort of numb in our surroundings, but when we get outside and visit with Mother Nature it reminds us of the struggle of life, the beauty of the present, and how getting wet might not be any fun, but being wet _together_ is.

# Control

## 2.

A loss of control is at the root of literally every challenge you will face in caring for YLO. The uncertainty and fear of the future that comes with Alzheimer's also creates an overwhelming amount of anxiety. Planning and preparing carefully can help reduce that anxiety for both you and YLO, so that you can maintain as much control as possible despite the disease.

When I work with families, I offer them more control. When I spend time with their loved ones, I ease the burden of constant care-giving for the family and allow them time to rest and focus on their own lives.

The work I do with my clients gives them more control, too. I help get them out of the house and build their confidence so that that they still feel independent and capable. I give them a break from their primary care-givers and, hopefully, a break from their Alzheimer's. I treat them normally and we do everyday things. When I take them home they often arrive acting like their old selves, feeling happy and a little more confident.

In this chapter I'll offer a few suggestions about how I think a simple rule of "safety first" can help you make a few difficult decisions regarding care. I also think that using existing routines and creating new ones can help tremendously with the amount of control you will have throughout the day. I believe simplifying and de-cluttering can ease some of YLO's confusion. To navigate your way through this I have an interview with Martha Stewart, or at least what I think she would say. I also have a few suggestions on YLO's own money management. I'll offer a few tips on how to avoid an argument and how to introduce "help" if there is resistance. Then I'll close this chapter imagining what AD might be like.

**Maybe some of this information can help you develop strategies for coping in your own situation.**

## Safety First

You can use a simple rule to approach every single question and decision you will face:

#1 Safety

#2 Budget

#3 Happiness

Safety is your number one responsibility as a care-giver. You are responsible as a wife, husband, son, daughter, brother, or sister to make sure YLO is safe. However, you are not responsible for their happiness. Happiness is still something to strive for, since a happier, healthier person can certainly cope with the challenges of AD more successfully than one who is unhappy, but happiness still and always comes after safety.

After safety, you have to make decisions that fit into your budget. If there isn't enough money, some things are not possible, and your decision is simple. After you've decided that safety is your primary concern, look at the kind of care that is necessary and stick to your budget when choosing the solution.

When you've figured out what will keep him or her safe, and what options you have within your budget, then you make your choice based on what will make YLO most happy.

## Happiness: Making the Effort to Find Joy

There is a big difference between getting out of the house just to get out of the house, and getting out of the house for something that is joyful. Your idea of a fun activity might not be YLO's idea of a fun activity. Things have changed quite a bit, and their interests might have changed too. Some guys become louder and more talkative and some become quieter. Some women might have enjoyed being with a room full of friends at one time but now that just intimidates them. We all change, but changes can be drastic when you have AD. Being able to recognize what makes YLO happy now as opposed to what used to make her happy can make a big difference when you are searching for enjoyable outings. I bet if you could get a clear answer from someone with AD you might hear, "Sure, an occasional big day is great! I love getting out. But being with my grandkids and my dog make me the happiest," or "I feel the best when I am out in the yard in the sun pulling weeds" or "I feel the happiest when I'm escaping to the movie theatre" or "walking in the woods by the river." And so on.

I have found that joy is a stronger emotion than anxiety. I know that it can be next to impossible for AD sufferers and their care-givers to feel joyful amid the anxiety and frustration, but it's still a worthwhile goal. Paying attention to what YLO enjoys and adjusting your approach accordingly will always help reduce anxiety for everyone. I'll give you an example.

During my weekly visits with a client in an assisted living facility, I noticed a lady who had advanced AD and was in bad shape. She cried all day. No one could figure out what was wrong or how to console her. One day I walked in and she had a baby doll in her lap. She wasn't saying anything but she actually had a smile on her face. I think she was a little overwhelmed (in a good way) by her responsibilities as a new mother. She was happy. One baby doll changed everything. Every time I see her now she is smiling. How simple! Complicated mixtures of medicines and tons of visits from family couldn't match the power of one baby doll. Stay aware of ways to bring joy to YLO (and be creative), so you can make the most of your time.

## Intense Emotions

Emotions can be amplified in people who have AD. They are losing a sense of control, losing memories, and might be reacting emotionally more and more every day. My clients might not remember what we did last week, but they will remember the feeling they had when we were doing it. If it was a particularly pleasant visit, the next visit will be even better because they will associate me with a good feeling. They might not remember the specifics, but they remember the way they responded emotionally to the experience. All of our memories are associated with emotions, so YLO is likely to have more intense moods than before. All the more reason to make the effort to find activities that will bring joy into their lives, since the feeling is what they will remember.

## Understanding

In the beginning, and certainly as the disease progresses, YLO might start to get a few words mixed up. They might forget what key goes where, how to use a computer, or may, for example, start to use a fork for ice cream. **It is frustrating** to watch someone you love forget the simplest of tasks, lose their train of thought in mid-sentence or, at times, seem as though they are not paying attention. Try your best to remember; it's the disease, not them.

I remember when Mom couldn't use her radio any more. It had been in her kitchen for years but she couldn't remember how to turn it on. I said to her over and over something like, "Mom, it's so simple, all you do is... I'm not sure why you can't grasp this?" I wish I could have that moment back. I wish I would have been a little more considerate and understanding of what she was up against.

YLO might be working hard trying to solve problems and searching for solutions to what we might think are simple tasks. He or she might also be working hard trying to conceal the disease. I believe if YLO knows, no matter what, they should never be embarrassed about being confused around you and that you are doing your best to understand why things have become more difficult for them, they might ask for help more often. If they ask for help, that gives everyone a little more control, relieves some of the stress you both probably share, and more importantly, might allow you to understand their world a little better.

## Routines, Repetition, Rituals and Habits

Since people with AD might not be creating too many new memories, if they can rely on the familiarity of old routines, life will go much more smoothly. With routines, they won't have to expend all their energy trying to remember what to do and how to do it, and they will be able to maintain much more control over their lives for much longer. This means your responsibilities as a care-giver might be easier.

**I was never a "routine-oriented" person, but that has helped me to understand how important routines can be to someone who is starting to struggle with everyday tasks.**

Also, the earlier you start introducing new routines, like recommended changes in diet and exercise, the more likely you are to have success. These *established routines* will be a huge help as Alzheimer's progresses. It can become more and more difficult to introduce anything new after a certain point and that is why it's so important to get a diagnosis as soon as possible, so you can start to set up these comforting and reliable routines for yourself and YLO.

I am able to maintain control with my clients, and help give them their own sense of control, through the use of routines and repetition. When my visits are predictable, my clients know what to expect which greatly reduces their anxiety. This helps me immensely by setting a relaxed tone for the day and our activities; if something happens to go wrong, things are much less dramatic.

If there are things to do and things to look forward to and my client has some control over his life by using these routines and repetition, I'm sure he will be happier. He might go to dinner every Friday night at his buddy's house or take one of his grandchildren to the movies every Saturday. Also, an afternoon walk with a friend (say... every Thursday) is a great way to spend time. I often help families plan out a week with a few consistent visits and activities with friends and family; consistency is crucial in keeping loved ones engaged and active. You might consider using a weekly calendar.

Making sure YLO has a consistent morning routine will set the tone for a structured day and will help you both get moving. He or she should wake up at the same time every day, and follow a schedule. *"Time to get up."* Pull the curtains, open the blinds and let the sun shine in. Make up the bed as soon as he gets up. Don't encourage a return back to bed for a *post-wake-up nap* – sleeping too much will add to YLO's overall confusion. Have breakfast, have him take his pills, shave (this is a good time to introduce an electric razor), take a shower, maybe walk the dog if he has one – have options for activities. In the afternoon, there's lunch, maybe a little TV, get out for a bit, a walk, and then maybe a nap. In the evening, there might be dinner out and a relaxing end to the day with a consistent bedtime.

**Establishing a morning routine that YLO can enjoy will be effective in reducing depression and anxiety. By using this routine, you may be able to keep YLO out of bed and back in the action.**

**Slippers off. Shoes on.**

Maybe a similar formula of keeping existing routines and using repetition might work for you.

## Heading Out

Making sure we follow a checklist every single time we leave the house is absolutely imperative for establishing and maintaining control. Before we leave I say, "House Key" – Check. "Cell Phone" – Check. "Wallet" – Check. Add to the list anything else YLO needs that will make him or her feel comfortable with the outing. Some of my clients can't leave the house without a compass, Chapstick, flashlight, dog treats, or a comb, and that's OK. Make sure they have everything they need to feel comfortable for the outing.

**Beneficial Habits Today Can Help with Tomorrow**

These include:

- A healthy diet with a wide variety of foods.

- Exercise routines with varied exercises and options to keep YLO moving.

- Socialization with options (visit friends and family, get out and go, participating in activities they have enjoyed their entire life and introducing new ones if possible.

If you incorporate these and build on them, when YLO reaches the later stages of AD you will have established some good solid routines that might help with the continuation of these activities. Some tastes for favorite foods might change, but the more varieties of food he likes, the longer you might be able to keep him interested in eating. It is the same with exercise and socialization. The more options you provide, the more opportunities there will be to keep YLO involved.

Over time, by using repetition, you might be able to introduce new activities. Here is an example: William wasn't interested in doing much of anything with anybody... and I was sure to be no exception. My plan: I would meet him on his walks at the YMCA. Slowly they became "our walks." After a month, William's wife told him to catch a ride home with his new walking pal – "me." A few weeks of this... "Hey William, on the way home let's grab lunch..." etc. It worked. I built "our routine" on one of his existing routines. This is why keeping the routines they have and **starting new ones** is so important. With no routines or any consistency in their lives, new experiences and going to new places might be too scary for them. When I was introduced to Paul two years ago, it was a difficult first few weeks. I started slowly with short visits. I used repetition: same routine, same roads, same restaurant and I waited months to gradually introduce new activities. Now we do Meals On Wheels every Wednesday, shoot pool (Paul is always stripes), and see movies. He wasn't up to doing anything (nothing, zero, nada) and now we are out and about. With most of the people I work with I can take them just about anywhere. I have taken the time to build trust and create a new neural pathway with routine and repetition.

Something to consider: Paul and I were introduced at the right time. If I walked into Paul's life today, it might be too late. I have been in a few client relationships where I tried to make a difference but it was just too late.

46

## Simplifying, Downsizing, and De-cluttering

Ignore this page if YLO loves clutter and always has. If they like to be surrounded by boxes, old newspapers and they have lived that way for years out of choice, it's part of their lifestyle. Let it be.

But, *"The things we own – really end up owning us."*

I have helped several of my clients downsize and get rid of clutter, junk, and trash. At first, they were reluctant – very reluctant. But just like everything I do, I took it slowly, starting with removing small amounts of stuff. I even lied and told them it was going into storage. I would bring in a few really nice storage boxes and a sheet of paper marked Storage Box #1. I'd tape the sheet to the box and we would go through piles of papers together. I'd put anything that was obviously trash (mailers, newspapers, old phone books, advertisements, packaging, etc.) into the boxes. Then I'd put the boxes by the door and, very carefully and discreetly, slip them out when my clients weren't looking. After a few months of this, the house or apartment looks better and the burden of all that junk is gone.

Even for a perfectly healthy person, it can be too overwhelming to look at all those boxes, old magazines and mounds of stuff and clutter. There is anxiety just from analyzing the amount of work that needs to be done. Some clients had lived their lives clutter-free, but with the onset of AD, things just started piling up. They stopped being able to differentiate between something meaningful and something trivial. Now, everything seems to be valuable: take-out menus, old newspapers, napkins... It's all part of losing your memory and trying desperately to hold on to anything that can remind you of things that have happened, what you did yesterday or last week.

If you can't get anywhere by working together to downsize and sort through the clutter, then I suggest that you go ahead and take care of it yourself. It's unfortunate to have to be a little sneaky, but removing small amounts over time is something that really will decrease anxiety for everyone.

**Imaginary Interview with Martha Stewart**

**Martha's Bio:** World's Greatest Homemaker.

Hello Martha,

> I hope all is well in the land of perfection. I have a few ideas about downsizing and getting rid of clutter for people who have dementia. I know that a certain amount of anxiety comes from their accumulation of stuff and their not being able to understand what is valuable and worth keeping and what is not. Also I'd like to save some time by limiting a few choices they have to make.

*(Martha) What a great idea, Henry! This will be so helpful for them.*

**Q. (Henry) What would you suggest to help men get dressed and ready for the day?**

A. *(Martha) Pick his favorite: seven shirts, seven favorite pants. Fourteen pairs of socks and seven pairs of underwear. Limit his choices. I bet if you just observed him he has probably already picked out his favorites. For example, the shirt he wears every day, get a few more like it. And get rid of the clothes he never wears or liked. Too many choices in the morning takes up too much time. Put the winter clothes up in spring and summer clothes up in the fall.*

*This is subjective but if he looks good he will feel good. If he knows that a particular shirt looks good on him, he will wear it. Don't touch the jackets. Men have a thing about their jackets – all of them. Even if they deny it.*

**Q. And how about the ladies?**

A. *The same. And for their shoes, get rid of the ones you know she won't wear. One nice pair for going out, one pair walking/exercise and one comfortable pair to wear around the house.*

**Q. Martha, what about kitchen and food items?**

A. *Clean out that fridge. Make sure that expired products are thrown out. Get rid of the three ketchups and that old jar of pickles. Two years is long enough. Keep it clutter free. Again, too many choices take up too much time. Some of that old food can be dangerous. You need to keep tabs on everything in there. Check for spoilage. I wish I could tell you to organize and streamline, but now is not the time to change things on your loved one. Leave the utensils, pots and pans where they have been for the last five years. But if you have small appliances like a bread maker, ice cream maker and espresso maker that are not being used any longer, get rid of them.*

Q. **My mom had three keys for her house: one for the front door, one for the side entrance, and one for the laundry room. She was carrying around three different keys and sometimes would get confused about which one to use. My uncle Roger picked up on that and changed out the locks. One key. Simple. No confusion. If YLO isn't driving any more, make sure his/her key chain has something on it. If there is a relic key chain that he bought at a souvenir hut, use it! YLO needs to stay in the habit of carrying keys as long as possible. Keys are control.**

A. *(Martha) Henry, you are so right about those keys!*

Q. **Pictures. Boxes of them. Unorganized and all over the place. What would Martha do?**

A. *I would create a storage box for each child or grandchild and start sorting them. You will feel great when it's done and enjoy reliving the memories. If the pictures are in a digital format, place them on a DVD so YLO can watch them on TV. Plus, I would place family pictures all over the house especially a few of the two of you together at the dining table. It's a great reminder.*

Q. **What about the garage or workshop?**

A. *Your father or husband use to build things. Now he has no interest. You might want to get rid of some of the dangerous tools like the table saw. Yikes! And speaking of dangerous, lock those guns up too – Goodness!*

> **Thanks Martha. I know you are busy and probably need to get out to your garden now to cut some fresh flowers for your dinner party tonight, so again thanks for your time.**

This is just an introduction to a few things you can organize and get rid of that will make things around the home a little bit "simpler" and less complicated. I bet with a good clean up and a haul to the recycle bin, you might even see a decline in YLO's level of anxiety.

## Control of Money

Money equals freedom, security, and power. Money is the essence of
control. When you think it's time to take the credit cards and cash away, be
mindful of what is really happening. You are taking away something more
than just money. Here are some suggestions that might help you navigate
this particular issue:

- Small amounts of cash can really make a difference. A $20 dollar bill,
  four $5 bills, and eight ones could be enough to keep YLO grounded,
  fill up their wallet, and allow him/her the ability to pay for a
  few things.

- Be practical about bank accounts. If YLO is your spouse, you might
  want to combine your accounts. In other cases, if you have Power of
  Attorney, you have the ability to manage YLO's accounts. If YLO uses a
  checkbook, invent a "safe place" to put it. Check-writing has the most
  potential for disaster, so take care to prevent as much as possible.

- Debit cards are a great option, since you can control the amount of
  money available in the associated account. Set a small limit and check
  statements routinely to monitor spending. If YLO can't remember the
  four-digit PIN or can't sign his name anymore, then it's time to take
  the card away.

- Credit cards are easy to use but can be more risky. Keep the limit low
  and carefully watch spending activity so that if anything happens you
  are aware of it immediately.

- My personal favorite solution is to use gift cards. One of my clients
  uses only gift cards when he goes out. His wife buys $25 American
  Express® gift cards, and makes sure that he has three or four in his
  wallet. He feels empowered and normal, he doesn't have to sign
  anything when he uses them, and his wife knows that his spending is
  under control.

- Tipping can cause some anxiety and prevent YLO from wanting to go
  out to eat. If he or she is paying the bill with cash and prone to over-
  tip, ask the waiter (preferably away from the table) to take twenty
  percent and bring the rest to you. Same if it's under. Ask the waiter to
  let you know how much it is under (again, away from the table). If he
  or she is paying with a credit card and has a hard time calculating the
  tip, then you take care of the tip to avoid this problem. The strategy
  is to say, "I know our server will appreciate a cash tip, so let me take

care of that." Just get into the habit of carrying a little cash for these situations.

## How to Speak Alzheimer's

I just read an article called "How to Communicate Better With Someone Who Has Early-Stage Alzheimer's." It said, "Slow down your speaking style. Enunciate your words to be as clear as possible. Use simple words and talk to them like you were talking to a young child."

Really?

I hope no one talks to me that way, ever.

I speak normally to everyone, every day, no matter what. I can get a little steamed if things aren't going as planned or I need to get someone's attention, but talking to someone with AD like they are a child is insulting. I talk to my clients as though there was no problem, no hurry to get anywhere. I keep things casual, with no emergencies. I stay cool, calm, and collected and I use positive reinforcement and encouraging words. I am gently coaxing when I have to be, and I reassure as much as is needed.

Try to communicate respectfully. I remember once when I was visiting Mom at the Lowman Home, a daughter was there visiting with her father. She kept asking him, "What color is my shirt, Daddy?", and, "How old are you, Daddy?" He had no idea how old he was or what color her shirt was. I wanted to say… "Hey lady, who cares what color your shirt is?!" I knew that her father was a paratrooper in WWII so I walked over and asked him, "Where were you on D-Day?" He said, "France." Then I asked, "Did you jump the night before?" He looked at me and said "Yes. 101st Airborne. Group Chicago. Flew over in a glider, rough landing but we made it!" He started talking up a storm. Even the staff came over. They were all amazed. This guy hadn't said much of anything for a few months, but when I engaged him in a normal conversation about a topic he knew about, he came to life.

Here are few short sentences that I use all the time when I'm communicating with my clients:

- You are right.
- That's it!
- Absolutely.
- I completely agree.

- You bet.
- I was thinking that, too.
- You could be right, but let's wait a bit.
- I was thinking the same thing.
- I couldn't have said it better.
- We always think alike.
- I'll tell you what – let's try it both ways.
- We can do it that way, too.
- You usually know what's best.
- I'm not sure about that – let's both think about it a little more.
- Last time we talked, you suggested we try this.

Usually when I'm in a social situation with a client such as visiting friends, restaurants, or a get-together, I try to include them in the conversations as much a possible. I try to direct the conversation toward the things that I know he or she will enjoy talking about.

As far as hearing the same question over and over or having to listen to the same story four times in ten minutes, here are several ways I "manage." I always want my clients to feel comfortable around me so I never say, "You just asked me that." I want my clients to continue enjoying conversations and I want them to feel as though they can say anything and that I'm listening. I just answer all their questions and listen to the stories. I can tune them out and politely say "yes" and nod, or help them along with their stories. Most of the time, I know the story so well I can tell it myself! Often I can redirect the conversation, but if I'm not able to do that, I just focus on being patient and respectful. Patience is more than a virtue when it concerns AD. Patience is **EVERYTHING.**

This is probably obvious, but try to be as calm and collected as you can. One time I spent a winter afternoon with one of my clients, William, who refused to unlock his front door even though he had his keys in his hands. He kept telling me that they wouldn't work. He never even tried them. We had been outside all morning. It was 35 degrees. We had come back from picking up hot food for lunch and William just wouldn't put the key in the lock. I had to take a step back and work on staying cool.

So, hold back, take a deep breath, use positive words and agreeable lines when you can, and you'll probably be able to avoid a showdown.

## Avoiding an Argument

I NEVER tell my clients that they are being unreasonable. Of course they are! They have Alzheimer's! With AD you could be dealing with someone who in some cases is losing their ability to reason, so the strategy is always to **persuade** or **redirect**.

One time my client Jack and I were in a movie theater. He stood up and said, "I need to go buy a car." Um... OK. So we walked into the lobby of the theatre. It had been burning him up for a few weeks that his wife wouldn't let him drive, much less buy a car. Now it was up to me, his pal. So I said, "I am in love with that new Chrysler too, but you have to get insurance first and they are always recalling a few of the models and..." I talked complete nonsense for five minutes and redirected the conversation until Jack was ready to get back into the movie and let go of the urgency to buy a car. I painstakingly recommended that we wait.

Instead of saying, "You are being unreasonable", be patient and don't push any buttons. Don't talk down or lose your cool. Take a part of what they are saying, use it to negotiate, and then take the time to persuade them. Use bits of the conversation to steer away from the topic and head in another direction – a friendly "direction." Avoid insults or confrontation. Let them think it was their idea and that you are working together. There are several books written on ways to communicate with someone who has dementia and trying and sum this up in two paragraphs isn't doing the subject justice, but I can say the more you do this, the more you will be able to figure out your own system. Eventually you will learn how to turn, twist and redirect the conversation.

Arguments are going to happen. Sometimes no matter what you say, even if it's the perfect thing, one of you is still going to lose control, or both of you are! Calm and collected doesn't work all the time. It might not even work some of the time for you, so I'll try to not be too ridiculous with my "advice" here. I don't want this to come across as naive thinking. Unreasonable people are stressful to be around and everyone snaps. Just try to remember, you are arguing with someone who has a brain disease and sometimes might be living in a different reality. When it's possible, make it seem like you are in agreement. You're not the boss; you're equal partners. My clients have a say in what we do, but I just negotiate with them until they want to do what I want them to do! If it seems like they have control over their decisions, they are happier and their level of anxiety is lower. Just like when dealing with the same question over and over – I know it can be exhausting, but the best way to cope is to try to lower the overall level of anxiety for YLO.

Do remember: Safety first. Then budget. Then happiness. Persuasion applies only in non-critical situations. With the car keys and bouncing checks, try persuasion first and then – take no prisoners.

## Anosognosia

Most of my referrals are for families who have tried to find help, but it just hasn't worked out. Based on my experience, my clients' attitudes can be a little more difficult to deal with than most. They don't think they need any help, have become less interested in leaving their home, won't cooperate, aren't interested in doing much, and **some won't acknowledge they have a problem.** These are all very real burdens to their care-givers. The irony is, it's those people with dementia who don't want to be a burden who are sometimes the ones that are the most difficult to care for.

This behavior (not acknowledging they have a problem) might be attributed to a common condition called anosognosia (a lack of awareness that one is impaired). It occurs frequently with people who have a mental illness, especially dementia. AD causes physical changes in the brain and researchers know that this damage can affect people's perception of their illness. Anosognosia might potentially be the reason someone will not accept an AD diagnosis.

I have clients that have what seemed to me a combination of both denial and anosognosia. I believe this combination is the main reason it can be so difficult to care for someone. **They don't think they need help.** The difficulty in caring for them is not because they are stubborn, trying to be independent or because they were raised a certain way. It's a symptom of the disease.

This is the most important reason I use an easy going approach and try to keep the anxiety and frustration levels as low as possible. I respectively try and gain their trust, use encouraging words and rely on structure and routine. These tools might allow you to introduce improvements in overall health, mood and happiness for both you and YLO.

## Talking to YLO About Alzheimer's

I rarely talked to Mom about AD. She didn't want to hear or talk about it. If we did talk about it, it was mostly in a joking manner. Having open and honest discussions can help but that depends on how accepting they are of the information. I work with some families that talk freely to their loved one about AD, and I work with families where there is no talk of it at all. Everyone processes it differently. Maybe it's because they have anosognosia? Maybe they are in denial? Whatever the scientific explanation is, most people I know can't confront the problem. **It's just too much to handle**.

I treat people the way I would want to be treated so I'm not so sure I would want to talk about it. That's the reason "ALZHEIMER'S" isn't written in bold red ink on the outside of this book. I'm not sure I would want to be reminded that I had a problem every time I glanced over at the book shelf.

I really like the way my client Tim deals with it. He is a Vietnam vet who was exposed to Agent Orange. He believes that is the reason his memory is not as good as it used to be. I think if I had AD, I'd like to think the way he does.

## Stretching the Truth

With AD there is no reasonable explanation sometimes for why someone says something or acts the way they do, so you have to be flexible. You have to be able to improvise, so you can make the best of your time.

And sometimes you have to lie.

When I get a call from a family member looking for my service it goes like this: I tell them a little about me and my experience with AD, but most of the conversation, I try to listen. I need to know as much as possible about the person I will be working with. If their loved one has acknowledged they have a problem, sometimes I introduce myself as professional trainer for Alzheimer's. If not, then we need to develop a plan for who I am going to be. I have to use a little trickery here because I work mainly with people who don't think they need help. Am I a volunteer from the VA or Meals On Wheels? Am I from their church, or maybe looking to join their church? Who I am (who I'm pretending to be) is important. This is how I have introduced myself several times:

> *"Hey Tim, I'm Henry. I do volunteer work down at the VA (Tim served in Vietnam). There is a program we have now where I'll come by once a week and we can go see a movie or hit a few golf balls. Whatever you might be interested in. It's free, because you served your country."*

*"Hello Chris. I was told you were a painter. If you would like, maybe you could help me with a class I was taking at Spruill Art Gallery."*

*"Hello Marie. I'm sure your daughter told you about me dropping by for a visit. I think it's wonderful that you would allow me to join you for Mass. I'm looking forward to learning about the Catholic faith and might consider joining."*

*"Hey Tom, I am a volunteer with Meals On Wheels. I'm looking for a copilot, someone who knows the area."*

I show up, introduce myself, and I know within the first ten seconds how the next three months are going to be. Are they glad to see me because he or she knows I'm there to get them out of the house? Are they suspicious and think I'm up to something? I act like there is no problem with their memory and get to work on gaining their trust. If the first time I met Marie I had walked in and asked her to go to lunch she would have thought I was crazy. So I told her I was interested in the Catholic Church and needed some guidance on maybe joining. She thought that was appropriate and it worked. You might find coming up with a few "schemes" will be a big help.

Some people welcome me into their lives in a minute and sometimes it takes a while to get where I want to go with this, but given enough time I can get there (if I am introduced early enough). After we get out and go a few times I expand our visit. "Let's get lunch on the way home." After a few more visits, "Can I see a few pictures of your family so I can put a face on everyone you have told me about?"

Once I am looking at pictures of kids or grandkids and listening to stories, I have gained a certain amount of trust. I have even taken my kids (accomplices!) over for a visit. Who can resist a one- year-old? Buzz Lightyear and The Sesame Street gang – Big Bird, Elmo, Burt and Ernie, are usually in my car, baby seats in the back, and that leads us to talk about most everyone's favorite subject who has kids..."kids!"

"What do I do for a living? I teach children how to play guitar. I start work at 3 pm when my students get out of school. I need to get out of the house and do something until then. That's why I'm with you."

As time goes on, they don't care who I am. They know fun and interesting are our pursuits and we get out of the house. I take people places they haven't been in years. We all (their families and I) work together in making a big difference in the lives of their loved ones. I take a lot into consideration. I design a specific day for each of my clients according to their interests. I'm also careful to find out by trial and error a few new things they enjoy doing. I don't look like *"help"* or act like *"care"*. My clients think I am a volunteer or they think I am the one who needs help, not them. I have an easygoing approach, and as I have said, I pretend there is no problem with anyone's memory. I am confident saying Let's Go wouldn't be as successful as it is if I didn't use one or two maybe even three very tiny white lies. A white lie, at the right time, can make all the difference in their world.

## Other Ways to Maintain Control

- I notice with most of my clients a certain normalcy can kick in when we get out and go. Not always, but when we are out on a nice day and on the way or coming back from doing something they enjoy, the general confusion may subside a little bit.

- I also understand you might be a bit apprehensive about taking YLO out because they might say something that doesn't make sense or they might say something that is a little too "interesting." I have a client that talks about his 45 pistol sometimes. At lunch at a downtown restaurant, he walked right up to a policeman, pointed at the officer's gun and said, "I have a 45." I immediately said, "And it's at home!"

Generally I have found that when I take my clients out and we interact with people, whether it be the staff at a museum, a waiter in a restaurant or just someone walking by, most people are incredibly nice and very understanding. Worrying about a few wild comments has never been enough for me to discourage anyone from getting out. If they are enjoying themselves, what's more important?

- In turn, don't try to fit too much into one day. I was hired by a family who ran their mother ragged with activities. Every time I turned around I was getting emails and calls about her appointments for the day. Her family was getting frustrated because she was refusing to go places she had always liked to go. So I said, "Hey gang, she sure talks a lot about Penny, her dog. Maybe you should set some time aside for her to just walk Penny." It turned out to become her favorite time. I know some of you want to fit everything in while you can because time is limited. I understand, but don't overuse activities and appointments. As always, be careful to consider what YLO really enjoys.

- A fifteen-minute wait if you have AD can seem like a month, so be aware that time is relative. That means planning ahead. How long will it take us to get ready? How long does it take to get there? I have learned that with some of my clients timing is crucial. If I have a good, thoughtful plan it makes for an enjoyable experience – and I always need to have a plan B.

- Having a plan B is essential: What if it is raining? What if it's 100 degrees outside? What if the movie starts in a half hour but he isn't even close to leaving the house yet? What if he is hungry but the plan was to have lunch in two hours, after the activity? What if he thinks he needs to go buy a car because his wife took his? This isn't easy! Have a plan B. You need to be able to improvise.

- Slow down. Don't be in a rush. It's all part of the "lowering anxiety plan." I have lived my life burning the candle at both ends but when you are around someone with dementia, you can't. You need to be as relaxed as possible around a loved one who has dementia. You mean a great deal to them, so take it easy. Stay calm, everything is A-OK. If you are relaxed and thoughtful, it most likely will reflect in YLO's attitude.

- Normal conversation: I engage my clients in normal conversation because they need to know that their thoughts and perspective are still valuable. Good topics for conversation can include politics, the news, religion, etc. Treat YLO like a friend, too, and confide your concerns and thoughts. Sharing some of your own worries and struggles will remind YLO that they can still be helpful to you, and might also help him or her to let down their guard and accept help from you.

- Talking about books with my clients has been an interesting strategy too. I'll pick up a book and ask, "Are you reading this? How is it?" I'll borrow books and then bring them back after a while, even if they can't read or comprehend what they are reading. I'll say, "The book you recommended for me was great!" Alzheimer's sufferers spend so much energy trying to conceal their memory problems. I continually work on giving them those tools back in any way I can so they feel like capable people who can still contribute, help others and take care of themselves.

- Try your best to understand a few behaviors: YLO is probably well aware that he/she is losing control over many decisions. My client

Bill knows this and sometimes he tries to take back some of that lost control. Occasionally, when we are almost out the door, Bill will put the brakes on and stall a bit. Just enough to let me know he is still in charge of a few things. It a small gesture with a big payoff. I get it. I understand and I welcome it. If Bill has more control, so do I.

- A safer environment gives you more control. Since YLO's safety is your number one concern, take a few precautionary steps to make YLO's home a safe environment (see Alz.org Caregiver Center/Home Safety).

- Driving: Taking the car keys away is a very difficult task. This one is tough on everybody. Cars represent freedom and independence. For men, cars are ingrained in our DNA; the lines, mechanics, and the loyalty to different brands. Here is usually what is recommended to the families I work with when it's time for their loved one to stop driving. I'm going to use my pal Allan (the dog lover) again as an example. Allan is furious. His wife says he is not allowed to drive any more:

Blame it on the doctor. Ask the physician to say "Allan, you need to take a driving assessment. Most people with what you have need to be observed to make sure you are still a safe driver." Allan is going to be angry, *but the doctor doesn't have to live with him.* Plus, many people think that whatever the doctor says is gospel – that is why it works.

When you have decided to take the keys, get rid of Allan's car immediately. Do not let it sit in the driveway. *Do not sell Allan's car to your neighbor!* Out of sight out of mind... hopefully.

Arrange to have a driving assessment for YLO (see Alz.org/In My Area/List of Driving Assessment Centers). This is what I say to my clients who think they should be allowed to drive: (Laws differ from state to state and even though I am making some of this up it seems to work.)

*If you fail the driving exam the DMV will be notified in 10 business days. The DMV will then notify your insurance company and cancel your policy. If you drive with canceled insurance and get in a wreck, especially if it's your fault, the other driver/pedestrian could get your house and empty the bank account. Your number one reason to not drive is to protect your family and all you have worked for.*

This is certainly about Allan's safety but more importantly, what about that kid on the bicycle that he didn't see?

- The TV remote, phones, DVD players, etc.: As AD progresses gadgets with buttons, dials and buzzers get difficult to use. Introducing new gadgets can be impossible! Here is an email from Cathy:

*William is very frustrated with the new remote to the TV, although it works just like the last one. We keep going over and over it and so far, he doesn't seem to grasp it.*

If YLO knows how to use the current remote control, don't switch on him or her. Same goes for all appliances, radios, DVD and CD players. If it's working – it's working. If you have to change then you might want to buy a simple to use remote control: On/Off. Volume. Channel. (See The Alzheimer's Store www.AlzStore.com). Also realize text message and emails might not be an effective way to communicate any more.

## Music

### "Listen to the Music" – Doobie Brothers[1]

I just skimmed an article about dementia therapy and music. "New Study – University so and so found that –

good music is good for you."

I hope they didn't spend a lot of money trying to figure that out.

When I'm driving around with my clients and one of their favorite songs comes on the radio, it's instant joy. It's a smile. A song can take us all the way back to that time when... So a good song will put you in a good mood? Of course it will. Music is therapeutic to people who have dementia – and that equals control, so cut on the radio! [2]

| | |
|---|---|
| **"Isn't She Lovely"** Stevie Wonder | **"I Walk the Line"** Johnny Cash |
| **"More Than a Feeling"** Boston | **"Philadelphia Freedom"** Elton John |
| **"Walkin After Midnight"** Patsy Cline | **"Moonlight Serenade"** Glenn Miller |
| **"Cruisin"** Smokey Robinson | **"Heart of Glass"** Blondie |

# Imagine What AD Might Be Like

I make my livelihood by caring for people who have Alzheimer's. I have to be creative, patient, and understanding of their experience in order to best help them. I've thought a lot about what it must be like to have AD, and I've had to put myself in my clients' shoes nearly every day. I've come up with a terribly simplified analogy for how I think it might feel, and how this feeling changes as the disease progresses.

**In the early stages:**

I bet it's a lot like being in London. They speak English in London, but with a very different accent. Some Londoners might as well be speaking Italian. So, you wake up in London and people are speaking differently. Crossing the street can be lethal. London is not a grid, so the streets are winding and unpredictable. Big streets and tiny streets intersect. You are in a confusing and fast-paced environment where your money isn't worth anything.

You grab your map, exchange some cash for pounds, and set out for a day of sightseeing. You are on your own. You can handle this, but there are times when you need some help finding things. You might need a little help ordering food or you might need help crossing the street... "Look right!" You're disoriented because it's all pretty overwhelming, but you manage to see a few sights. You eat some authentic fish and chips and get back home safely. You are a little nervous because what used to be easy seems like it takes a lot more energy.

**In the moderate stages:**

This time you are in Paris and you can't speak French. The map is in French too. What a beautiful city but it's tricky getting around. You can see the Eiffel Tower but can't quite figure out the right roads to take. Some words are familiar and you can use gestures (pointing, thumbs up) to ask a few simple questions. Oui? But speaking with anyone is very difficult. You walk into a restaurant... oh my, how frustrating! You are hungry but you haven't a clue how to order anything. You need help getting around and even communicating.

**In the advanced stages:**

You are now in Moscow, where not only do you not speak the language but you can't even recognize the Cyrillic alphabet to read signs. The circular street pattern in the city is completely confusing. Based on your experience in Paris, you are anxious that you won't be able to get around, and you are afraid to even get out of the hotel. Asking for help is hard, ordering food is impossible, and the food is strange. You don't understand what's on TV. You need help doing just about everything.

This is terribly simple. I know, but consider this when you might be having a problem taking someone who has AD out of the house. I always try to be a good tour guide.

Rx

# 3.

Clearly, medical care is a major part of managing Alzheimer's. If you haven't seen a neurologist, now is the time. Neurologists and psychiatric professionals play a critically important role in YLO's future. The attention, awareness, and research surrounding this disease has given us numerous options for medications that can help tremendously with quality of life, mood, and brain functioning. In fact, in some studies, widely available antidepressants have been shown to counter the effects of dementia on the brain. Our primary goal is to maximize quality time we have with our loved ones, so along with working on exercise, nutrition, and socialization, a commitment to the pursuit of proper treatment is imperative.

**Interview with Dr. Lah**

Hello Dr. Lah,

You have been instrumental in helping me start Let's Go, and I can't thank you enough. Your referrals and your trust in my program and what I'm striving to accomplish have been so beneficial to the success we have achieved thus far.

Bio: James J. Lah, M.D., Ph.D. Director, Emory Cognitive Neurology Program, Memory Assessment Clinic, Atlanta, GA.

> Q. **(Henry) What is your initial advice regarding medical care for a family who thinks a loved one might have Alzheimer's?**
>
> A. *(Dr. Lah) It is critical that a proper evaluation be completed and accurate diagnosis made as early as possible. There are several reasons for this. The prospect of Alzheimer's is terrifying for most people, and many patients and families do not want to confront the frightening prospect. The situation is similar to a person confronting a diagnosis of cancer, and complicated by the fact that*

*Alzheimer's erodes the ability to come to grips with the implications of disease. Nevertheless, I feel strongly that each person deserves the opportunity to confront the challenge and decide how he or she wishes to respond. Delaying diagnosis or being vague about what is happening makes this more difficult for the person as symptoms progress.*

*A related consideration is that establishing a diagnosis and understanding its implications may help patients and families avoid potentially disastrous consequences stemming from unaddressed symptoms. For example, we have had a number of families who have had to deal with financial problems because of poor decisions made by the patient or because an unscrupulous individual exploited a vulnerable person. If one is aware of the potential hazards, safeguards can be put in place to avoid such tragedies.*

*Our current treatments are limited to "symptomatic" drugs. By this, I mean that the drugs alleviate Alzheimer's symptoms but do not alter the course of the disease. An analogy for this is the use of pain medications for a progressive joint deterioration (e.g. your right knee). Ibuprofen or acetaminophen may help ease the pain, but as the joint continues to deteriorate, the pain will recur and we achieve less effective pain relief from the same dose of drug. Regardless of the point in Alzheimer's disease at which current medications are given, they afford the same amount of modest symptom relief. This can be viewed as extending a phase of illness or turning back the clock (by perhaps 6 months) through the symptomatic effects of the drugs. Subsequently, although the drugs continue to work, the disease progresses and the patient becomes sicker. My view is that the 6 or 12 months of symptomatic benefit is of greater value if it extends a period of milder symptoms than if we wait and apply the drugs at a point when symptoms have progressed and quality of life has degraded.*

*Lastly, while our current therapies are limited to symptomatic drugs, research efforts are squarely focused on finding treatments that will help to delay onset or slow progression of disease. It is almost certain that these "disease-modifying" treatments will be more effective and more beneficial if applied as early as possible in the course of Alzheimer's disease.*

**Q. When a loved one is diagnosed with Alzheimer's, what questions should families ask when first seeking help from a neurologist?**

A.  *The first step is to make sure that the diagnosis is clear. Too often, I see patients who have been given rather vague diagnoses such as dementia or memory loss, rather than a specific diagnosis of Alzheimer's disease. Brain diseases, such as stroke or cerebrovascular disease, front-temporal dementia, Lewy body dementia, and others, can all cause memory loss or dementia. Other medical or psychiatric conditions, such as depression, sleep apnea, hypothyroidism, vitamin B12 deficiency, and others, can cause or contribute to memory loss and dementia symptoms. The neurologist should evaluate each of these possibilities, and address them appropriately in the overall management of the patient.*

*Since we are limited in our current options for treating patients with Alzheimer's, I always look for opportunities to "add by subtraction." There are many drugs in common use that can worsen thinking abilities and exacerbate symptoms. These can include drugs that a person has been using for many years. Although the drug may be the same, the person has changed. For example, sedative-hypnotic drugs such as diazepam (Valium), lorazepam (Ativan), or alprazolam (Xanax) may have been prescribed to help manage mild anxiety symptoms. This was a common practice for many years (remember the Rolling Stones' song "Mother's Little Helper"?). Unfortunately a drug that may have worked great for you when you were 45 may have very different effects on you when you are 75. Your liver is different, your brain is different, and the drug may now adversely affect how your brain works. This may be true for a healthy person and is a greater concern for someone with Alzheimer's disease. Be sure to ask if there are medications that may be having a harmful effect, and eliminate them whenever possible.*

*In addition to finding out about medications, address practical issues. Given the stage of illness and severity of symptoms, what precautions should be taken? Does she require more supervision? Can he still drive safely? These are very difficult questions, and not all physicians will be comfortable addressing them. The guiding principle in all such instances is to maintain as much independence and dignity as possible while recognizing that he or she may not always accurately recognize limitations and safety concerns. Clinical experience teaches us that establishing routines of stimulating activities is helpful for patients and for care-givers. Find solutions that work best for your family. Ask and find out about sources of education and support for the patient and loved ones. If the physician cannot provide this information, seek it elsewhere through sources such as the Alzheimer's Association, the Emory Alzheimer's Disease Research Center, and the National Institute on Aging, all of which maintain reliable information on their web sites.*

**Q.** **Through my experience I've seen that AD really does affect everyone differently. Is there an explanation for why AD's effects are so widely varied?**

A.  *There is not an easy explanation, but your observation is certainly accurate. We tend to think of Alzheimer's as something of a monolithic entity, but it isn't. There are sufficient commonalities in pathology, biochemistry, and genetics that we can reasonably identify a group of individuals as having the same disease. However, each person represents a unique combination of genetic factors and life experiences, and there is an unfathomably complex set of interactions between them. We know for instance that some genes can increase or decrease specific types of Alzheimer's pathology in certain parts of the brain, and variable involvement of different parts of the brain may cause one person to have more language difficulties while another has more problems with visuospatial abilities. There has been a lot of recent interest in traumatic brain injuries suffered by professional athletes because we believe that those events increase the likelihood of developing Alzheimer's and other degenerative brain diseases. Depending on which areas of the brain may have been injured, these past events may affect the future manifestation of Alzheimer's symptoms. Each of us is unique largely because of differences in the development of our brains and the changes that accumulate in them through a lifetime of experience. In a way, I suppose it should be expected that when a disease like Alzheimer's assaults that repository of our selves, the injury will result in a set of symptoms that are unique to each affected person.*

Thank you, Doctor Lah. You have been a tremendous help and I know everyone reading this will have a much better understanding of this disease. I would also like to recognize Allan Levey, MD, PhD, Janet Cellar

DNP, PMHCNS-BC, Stephanie Vyverberg APRN, NP-C. I'd like to give a special thank-you to Susan Peterson-Hazan MSW, LCSW.

Dr. Lah represents everything good about modern medicine. My clients who are his patients know and tell me that they are being given the best care available. I believe this to be true. I felt his sincerity and honesty in the interview was the most refreshing and interesting I have heard on the subject. He is indeed an asset to his patients, and his research is vital to one day finding a cure for Alzheimer's.

## Medication

I became overwhelmingly aware of the miracle of medications when one of my clients, Scott, became increasingly delusional and had to be admitted into a psychiatric hospital. His disease had advanced and we weren't sure if he'd be able to live at home any longer. He was observed for a week and they reviewed the medications he was already taking. A new combination of antidepressants and anti-psychotic drugs was prescribed for him. This new combination worked so well that Scott was able to return home and we were able to continue our visits and activities. I am a believer. I have seen it work, and I want you to know there is hope. These drugs have given my clients and their families the precious gift of more quality time together.

Not to go on too long but this is IMPORTANT. Certain medications can have a profound and positive impact on every one's life: Just this year I had a client (whose bags were packed – ready to go to memory care) but one last ditch effort with a new medication and he is still home, happy and his family is not (yet) writing a huge check every month for assisted living. One pill can be a game changer.

## Antidepressants

Medications can provide a better life for patients who have Alzheimer's. What I have noticed is that it's the antidepressants and the anti-delusional/anti-psychotic drugs that make the biggest difference. For my clients these medications play a critical role in helping them get out and go and enjoy life again. Simply, they can work. Sometimes it's an ongoing process for the doctors to come up with the right medications, the right combination and the right dosage, but when the parameters are met this seemingly small success can often offer much more control for both you and YLO.

Talk to your doctor about antidepressants and see what she or he might recommend.

## Delusions

de·lu·sion

di'loōZHən/noun  plural noun: delusions

1.  An idiosyncratic belief or impression that is firmly maintained despite being contradicted by what is generally accepted as reality or rational argument, typically a symptom of mental disorder.

I don't want to alarm you too much here. YLO might never have delusions, or at least the kind we all associate with dementia... like in the movies. I struggled through a few AD related movies. Honestly, I have yet to see even part of one where an actor actually captured what AD is really like. It's impossible. I just think it's important for you to know that some dementia patients (not all) may become delusional at some point in the progression of the disease, **usually in the later stages**. If that occurs, it's better to be prepared. It's also important to realize that these delusions are very real situations for these patients.

A delusion can be as simple as being confused, just for a moment, about where you are or what you are doing. It might last as long as a heartbeat, but it can be a little scary. It would be for me. I always try and help the person to get their footing, so I might subtly remind them where we are, what we are doing and say "Everything is A-OK." When I'm with someone **in the later stages of AD**, then, of course it can be more difficult to help them get their footing. His/her delusion might consist of working out a problem, or working out various problems, all at once – "What in the world is going on?" If that's the case, I'll try and redirect and change the subject. I might introduce something for them to concentrate on like a picture or bring up a favorite story or memory of theirs. If the delusion is a happy memory, something fun and exciting, I might even roll with it. If they think they are at the train station waiting to leave for a trip, I might say, "How exciting! Would you like to get something to eat before you leave?"... and then I try to gently welcome them back to "here."

Why a person with AD acts the way they do is a difficult question to answer, but obviously part of the brain isn't properly functioning. Other factors could be their own personalities and history and since the brain is "your mind" there are probably a few unknowns. Sometimes, the delusions can be caused simply by being forgetful and confused.

Several of my male clients hide their wallets. Once or twice a month we have to check a few places throughout the house before we leave because a wallet has been misplaced. Even though they are no longer allowed to drive, they are still protective of their driver's license, so they hide it. They are trying to hold on to anything that grounds them. Something they have in their back pocket for 50-plus years is certainly very important to them. Even though this is delusional behavior, I can understand.

Often delusions can be manageable but sometimes they can become uncontrollable. You and YLO might be strolling along, you might have become accustomed to a few of his "quirky" behaviors, and then out of the blue a new behavior challenge appears. *"He has never done this before!"*

With unmanageable and aggressive behavior, you honestly don't have many options. If he or she is showing signs of violent behavior, consult your doctor immediately. If they are dangerous to themselves and possibly you, then it's time for YLO to be observed by professionals.

But what if there isn't aggressive behavior? What if they just won't leave their room because they are in a "meeting" and they don't want to be disturbed? Maybe they haven't eaten or slept for some time. I help families who struggle with situations like this and since it's not an emergency, it can be even more difficult for the care-giver to know what to do. It's purgatory. This is why it's so important to have a dialogue with YLO's physician. You might also consider a "psychiatric evaluation" (more on Pg.141 First question) where doctors can observe YLO over a few days. The right medication at the right dose can make a huge difference.

Call your doctor and discuss YLO's behavior IN DETAIL when these situations occur. Give verbatim statements and behaviors. The more information you can give your doctors, the more they can help you with treatment decisions. Here are few suggested questions for your doctor in case you start to notice some delusional behavior.

1. *Here are some examples (a list) of how my husband/wife/mom/dad has acted lately. Are these delusions? What are the primary causes?*

2. *What types of drugs have had the most positive effects on patients who are delusional? Which ones do you think might help us?*

3. **When these delusions can't be controlled at home, what steps do I need to take? What are the procedures for admission into a psychiatric hospital? Who do I call? Who makes the referral? How will I know when I need to do this?**

## Sundowning

At about 4:00p.m. some people with dementia can start to become a bit "active." They call this Sundowning. Again, this doesn't happen to everyone but it happened enough to call it something. It makes sense to me. The moon is replacing the sun which might add to some of the anxiety already present.

This is a helpful website:

National Institute on Aging
www.nia.nih.gov/alzheimers/publication/sundowning

## Side Effects

I received a text from Carrie, my client Steve's wife. She said, *"Steve might not be as energetic this morning because they switched him to a different AD medication. With the one he was on, I noticed some improvement with his memory but the side effects were too bad."*

You might run into this. I did.

These medicines can work wonders, but it can be terribly confusing to know what to do if YLO is experiencing uncomfortable side effects from prescribed medications. I know exactly how that feels. My Mom's sisters, Mary Beth and Evelyn, and I took her to see a neurologist in Augusta, Georgia. He put Mom on a medication that sometimes gave her an upset stomach. She felt queasy nearly every other day. I had a difficult time deciding what to do. When I asked for advice from her prescribing physician, I wasn't able to get his attention. During that time, I kept Mom on the medication because I thought that the experts knew best. I was overwhelmed and afraid and was falsely convinced that this medicine was our only chance to save Mom's memory. Ultimately, I learned a lesson: Some healthcare providers are much better than others.

While Mom was coping with the nausea her medicine was causing, I was planning to take her to see her hero, Garrison Keillor. Mom loved the radio, and I grew up listening to the stories on "A Prairie Home Companion" with her on Saturday nights. It was always Frick and Frak in the morning and Garrison in the evening. So I got two tickets to the Fox Theatre in Atlanta, made special dinner plans, and waited for the big day. Her friend Don was planning to bring her to Atlanta for the show, but three days before,

I talked to her on the phone and she said she felt too sick and she just couldn't go.

We both cried over the phone. I realized that this drug I thought would improve her life was robbing us of precious time together, time we could never get back. Mary Beth informed Mom's personal physician of the situation and he immediately told us to take her off whatever was making her feel so bad and put her on something new. We never went back to Augusta.

If YLO is taking a medication that causes side effects that limit his or her functioning and enjoyment of life, there is no benefit. The drug may be slowing some of the progression of the Alzheimer's, but living with unbearable side effects is much more damaging than the disease itself. My mom and I lost valuable time, all because I didn't know it was OK for her to stop taking her medication and try something else. If you find yourself in this situation, don't allow YLO to suffer from side effects when there are so many other options out there. Remember that the ultimate goal is to help YLO make the most of every day.

# Family Business

# 4.

As soon as you've gotten a firm Alzheimer's diagnosis, it's going to be important to address the business that your family will need to handle. There are numerous and difficult decisions regarding finances, legal details, and funeral planning. There is also the issue of working with your family members to define care-giving responsibilities and create strategies for cooperating and bringing out the best in each other despite the challenge you are all facing together.

I knew with my mother's dementia, I was going to need a lot of legal and financial advice, and I was lucky enough that my Aunt Mary Beth and Don, Mom's great friend, set up an appointment for us with a good elder law attorney. I didn't really know what elder law was about, but it was actually the best step we could have taken for understanding and direction. Meeting with her reduced our deep anxiety about money, financial planning, and all of those "details." Elder law is a special area of legal practice that addresses power of attorney (as in, who gets to make decisions) as well as things like wills, living wills, and financial planning for the medical care you choose for YLO.

Here is a list of what elder law attorneys can assist families with: Asset protection, disability, estate planning, guardianship, long-term care, Medicare and Medicaid, mental health issues, power of attorney, retirement and pensions, Social Security, management of estates, trusts, and wills.


**Interview with An Elder Law Attorney**

I talked to a great elder law attorney in Atlanta and asked him some questions that might help guide you as you begin to address your legal and financial questions.

**Bio**: Philip Erickson concentrates his practice on estate planning, probate, and general commercial law. He is a member of the Florida and Georgia Bars, and the Elder Law and Estate Planning sections of the Atlanta Bar Association. Has worked for the Volunteer Income Tax Assistance (VITA) program since 1996.
http://www.okelleyandsorohan.com/Additional%20Areas.html

Hello Phil,

I really appreciate your help with these questions.

### Q.   (Henry) What is POA? Power of Attorney

A.   *(Phil) The financial power of attorney enables the person you select to act on your behalf. The powers can be limited by not initialing specific powers listed on the form, and you may elect to only have the powers take effect after an event or contingency occurs, such as incapacity as determined by a doctor. This financial power of attorney may be revoked at any time. This form prevents your family from having to go to court and have a guardian or conservator appointed to manage your property and affairs in the event that you should become incapacitated.*

*The durable medical power of attorney for health care enables the person selected to make health care decisions for you in the event of your incapacity. This could be important in the case of a medical emergency. The power is broader than the powers granted in a living will. For example, the health care power of attorney, just like a living will, may allow for the withdrawal of food and water. This can be very important, for example, if an individual is brain dead, but can be kept alive through the administration of food and water. The health care power of attorney also would allow you to place your loved one in an assisted living facility if the need arises. This form is also fully revocable.*

*Your decision to use this document is a very important one and you should think carefully about what financial decisions you want your Agent to make for you. The "Agent" is the person you give power to handle your financial affairs. The "Principal" is you. With this document, you can give your Agent the right to make all financial decisions or only certain, limited decisions. For example you can allow your Agent to handle all your financial affairs, including the power to sell, rent, or mortgage your home, pay your bills, cash or deposit checks, buy and sell your stock, investments, or personal items, or you can allow your Agent to handle only certain or specific financial affairs such as to pay your monthly bills.*

**Q. My Aunt Mary Beth and I worked well together regarding Mom's power of attorney but I have been involved in a few situations where POA was a bit contentious. With a larger family, things can get complicated about who obtains POA. When is the best time to settle who will have POA and who will be a 2nd POA?**

A. *No easy answer here, as every family is different – but often naming two people as co-agents helps prevent things from progressing too far without compromises and discussions taking place.*

**Q. What is the most asked question you get from families?**

A. *How to protect assets if a parent goes into a long-term care facility, and how the spouse can protect him/herself.*

**Q. Do you have any advice for a family that knows they need to see an elder law attorney but can't commit just yet?**

A. *If price is a concern, they should at least get powers of attorney in place to hopefully avoid guardianship and conservators being needed if something happens. This is a low cost start and helps avoid some of the most common problems.*

**Q. What is a living will?**

A. *The living will/advanced directive provides for the withdrawal of life-sustaining procedures in the event you become terminally ill and death is imminent. The living will thus allows you to arrange for a dignified death without prolonged suffering in the situation where the application of life-sustaining procedures would only serve to postpone the moment of death. By executing a living will, you may be assured that your wish regarding life-sustaining procedures will be honored in the absence of your ability to give directions should such a situation arise. A properly executed living will also relieves loved ones of the heavy burden of responsibility concerning whether to discontinue life-support procedures should such a decision be required. This document is also revocable.*

Q.  **Do you have any advice for preparing for the end? What are common mistakes that people make?**

A.  *By far, the most common mistake is doing nothing at all – and this causes more problems when the person is still alive, as someone needs to assist them in managing their affairs. If they don't have a will, probate is not that much more difficult – it just takes longer and you have no say where things go, it must go to the relatives named in the Code.*

**Thanks Phil. I know these decisions are the most important for the well-being of the spouses and/or the children. Your information should be very helpful.**

When we took Mom to see an elder law attorney, I remember feeling so much better after the visit. In two hours, I knew the possibilities as far as her long-term care. We now had direction and some confidence that we really needed. I remember walking out of our elder law attorney's office thinking, "Thank goodness we just did that." Aunt Mary Beth agreed 100%. It was incredibly informative. Questions answered. Anxiety reduced.

"OK... we can do this."

**Helpful Websites**

www.alz.org  (Look under Financial and Legal Planning).
www.longtermcare.gov (About Long-Term Care insurance and advice).

**Early Onset Alzheimer's**

My mom was diagnosed with Alzheimer's when she was 64. That is young. Early Alzheimer's disease is sometimes referred to as early onset or younger Alzheimer's. This type of dementia is distinct because its symptoms begin before age 65. I had always assumed that this form of AD was more aggressive, but since there are so many difficulties in diagnosing early onset Alzheimer's, researchers are uncertain about how fast it advances. I believe it has the perception of being more aggressive because it affects people at an earlier age, striking patients before retirement, sometime even while kids are still living at home. The patient might even be in the process of helping out their elderly parents. Simply, it wreaks more havoc on the family and is more destructive financially because it happens so early in life. Recently, I was hired by a family to work with Ed. He just turned 51.

Access to resources is vital.

## Helpful Websites

www.alzforum.org (Look under Early-Onset Familial AD).

www.alz.org (Look under Life with ALZ/If You Have Younger-Onset AD).

## When You Need Their Co-operation

Talking to YLO unemotionally can help when you need co-operation, especially regarding financial decisions. If you can remove the rhetoric, be blunt, direct and informed (or sound informed!) you might have an easier time convincing YLO what needs to be done. The trust you once shared might be a bit shaky due to the symptoms of the disease, so take the time to show them the facts and figures and, when it is possible, try and include them in the decision making.

## Just Getting Along

*"Most parents would be thrilled that their children are working in harmony in making decisions together and caring for their parents. It would bring the greatest joy for a mom and dad."*

The Reverend Howard Maltby, who married my wife and me in Columbia, South Carolina, in 2003.

In a dream world, everyone in the family pitches in, helps face the difficulties, sets aside personal issues, and works together for the greater good. All the decisions are made on time, everything gets signed and delivered, and everyone agrees in the end...

*and I haven't worked with a single family that was prepared for Alzheimer's. There is always stress, sadness, confusion, tension, and difference of opinion. Some families work together and get through it, but I've seen other families completely fall apart. Brothers and sisters stop talking, mothers get angry, grief paralyzes siblings and spouses. This whole experience puts a tremendous strain on any family. If you are seeing things like depression, fatigue, anxiety, and panic in yourself and/or your family members, don't think you are alone.*

I also have to mention what I call "Out of Towner Syndrome." This usually occurs when a family member that lives out of town thinks they understand the situation better than the ones who live close by or "in the same house." I could get into a whole lot of trouble here but I'll just say – in most of the families I work with that don't get along – it's a common theme. Understanding Alzheimer's is "on the job training" so there is something to be said about being present.

At this point in time, you are all hopefully thinking clearly enough so that you and your family can get together and create your own personal plan to deal with the family struggles you'll face together. On the following page is a document, written like a contract. At some point, you need to sit down together and do your best to focus on practical planning and considerations, and potential pitfalls that might arise along the way. If at all possible, this meeting should be in person with open and honest conversation and early enough that the person with AD can participate.

This document is designed to give you a reference tool for making decisions later on when you feel completely overwhelmed. When the time arrives to make decisions, everyone can look back at this document and say, "Three years ago we all shook hands and agreed on this. Everyone has a copy. Now it's time for action."

The following are six questions, and if you can answer all six, then personally I think you are in great shape for the challenge that lies ahead. Send copies to everyone involved and ask them to have a get-together when everyone has had time to think about the questions. Have a discussion and try to find some common ground needed to advance the cause. A little heated discussion now might save a total breakdown in the future.

It might.

## Initial Questions for Your Family Agreement

1. Finances:

☐ Have you talked with an elder law attorney?

☐ Have you talked with your siblings about total assets? Income? What each means as far as the future and health care needs and options?

2. Power of Attorney:

☐ Have you discussed who gets power of attorney?

☐ Will you have any co-agents?

3. The Will and Inheritance:

☐ Is there a will? Has everyone read it? Are there any questions? Has it been discussed among everyone involved?

4. Living Will:

☐ Does everyone understand what a living will is?

5. Working together:

☐ Will you accept advice from doctors, counselors, and other professionals, support groups, family members, friends? Will you work together to find these advisors?

6. Considering YLO in every decision:

☐ Will you make each and every decision based on what YLO would have wanted when he or she was of sound mind?

This family agreement is for families who can put aside past differences and can concentrate on the task of caring for a parent. If you are in a family who can't get in a room and discuss a few options or choices about the care of a parent without a lawyer or the police around, then this is probably not for you.

## Money

*"Money is freedom."*    Sandra T. Watts

My mom was what they call "a penny pincher." She was frugal and thrifty. When she was sixteen, her dad died (suddenly at 43) and the family fell on some rather lean times. Not "hard" but lean. With no income, Grandmother needed to be around family to help them get back on their feet, so they moved back to South Carolina. That very early-in-life experience and heartbreaking disappointment introduced my mom to the idea of saving for the future.

Mom was a secretary for South Carolina Educational Television, the local public PBS station, for ten years, and was a secretary at the University of South Carolina. She saved her money and bought a house. She was saving for her retirement AND in case something happened. She had everything prepared. Her will, living will. Funeral arrangements. Every consideration was taken care of. She even had a personal note in her will that was hilarious:

---

May 6, 1997  "Tying up loose ends before Don (her friend) and I leave for London."

Henry,

Here are some papers that you don't need to look at unless, God forbid, something bad happens to Don and me. I want to be prepared, just in case! You know me – It's my early Girl Scout Training. Enclosed are:

1. A copy of my instructions for organ and tissue donation. 2. Declaration of a desire for a natural death: Uncle Roger is the agent with power to enforce. I knew he'd like that job. 3. Travel insurance information: If I should happen to meet my maker (or just another car) on one of those narrow winding roads I've heard so much about, I do not (underlined) want my body boxed up and shipped home. Whenever and wherever I go to my reward, I want what is called "direct cremation". The travel insurance company should provide a really nice (maybe mahogany) box for my ashes for the journey. I'm sure they will be thrilled to not have to shell out for the huge expense of the alternative.

OK, that's enough of this kind of talk. Oh, one more thing – when the time comes I do want Henry's band Spectralux to play and my sisters to sing "Amazing Grace" at my service.

---

Everything was in place for us. She planned for the future, for which I am very grateful. My mom was very thoughtful and was wise enough to know that things might not work out as we plan them and that life can take a turn for the worse at any minute. She did not want to put me in a situation where I'd be taking care of her. That was very important to her. She loved me so much that she had the foresight to plan for "our" future. That's what love is.

I know talking about money is rude to do in public. I just want to give you a few numbers so you can judge for yourself a little bit about where you are.

After Mom was diagnosed, the elder law attorney told us that certain things needed to happen: We needed to live frugally, she needed to live on her own and to avoid assisted living as long as possible and hopefully stay relatively healthy. If this happened she might have enough in assets to get her through. If she outlives her money (that might be a possibility if she is in a nursing home for a long time), then you could be in trouble. "You might want to investigate which Homes have "Medicaid beds." I can't go into too much detail here, which is why you need to talk to an elder law attorney. Mary Beth and I agreed that we needed to look for a Home where they accepted Medicaid in case Mom did run out of money.

That was Columbia, South Carolina, from 2005 to 2008. Now, I'll bring you to today in Atlanta. I would think the price for assisted living in Atlanta would be on the high end. Here you can find a great assisted living home from $2,500/month and up. No doubt that $2,500.00 is a lot of money, but for room and board, safety, security and peace of mind – I think it's good value, especially compared to the cost of 24/7 in-home care. When it's time for skilled care/nursing, you are looking at more money. A lot more. I have seen as high as $9,000.00 a month. That kind of money would have wiped Mom out financially in less than a year. Gone. So, if your total assets are under a specific number and there is no Medicaid bed, what do you do? You worry.

My mom had the foresight, vision and thoughtfulness to plan for the future in case of an emergency. An emergency arose: Alzheimer's. She had to retire earlier than expected. She lived at home for as long as she could. We moved her into an assisted living home that she could afford and financially we made it.

I suppose this is as a good a place as any to talk about funerals!!!

**Interview with Daisy**

Through this interview with Ms. Harman, I hope to lower the level of anxiety for a care-giver who is facing the often frightening experience of planning the funeral for their loved one. By providing some pointers or a guide for you to begin preparations now, it won't be as scary and you won't feel so overwhelmed when the "time" actually arrives. I remember the staff at Dunbar Funeral Home that Mom had chosen was so helpful, and they carried out every detail to perfection. It was such a relief to know that Mom had made all her arrangements and that when the time came, everything would be in place. I didn't have to make any major decisions at a time when I was mourning her loss and not thinking as clearly as I normally would. When forced to make decisions while you are grieving, you are more apt to overspend or overcompensate for the loss. In some instances, you find it difficult to make a decision at all.

Daisy Harman is a Funeral Director at Caughman-Harman Funeral Home in Lexington, South Carolina, which has been in business since 1966. She is friend of my stepmother Martha and attends the church that my family attends and where my friend, the Reverend Howard Maltby, is the Rector. She is a calm presence who meets with families and provides guidance and assurance as they either plan their own funerals or others. Daisy is a true friend, as gracious and welcoming as they come.

Hello Daisy,

I appreciate your taking the time to talk with me about preplanning funeral arrangements and why it is so important to make these arrangements in advance.

**Q. (Henry) Why should I preplan a funeral?**

A. *(Daisy) It gives you the comfort and peace of mind that you have taken care of this, and your family will not have to make those decisions at a very stressful and emotional time. Another benefit is you can pay for it ahead and lock in the price. Some people say "well, it's just hard for me to do that," emotionally I guess, but I say consider it an act of business, as you would go to a lawyer to make a will, health care, or power of attorney, or any other directives regarding end-of-life planning. Sometimes that helps. Do it for your family. The main reason people come in is so their children won't be faced with these decisions.*

**Q. One of the main reasons for our interview is to lower the level of anxiety that a family might have in coming to see you to prepare.**

A. *I find that when people come in to do this ahead of time, when they leave they actually say, "You know, you made us feel so comfortable, we really enjoyed meeting with you, and we feel so much better. Our spirits are just lifted because we came in and did this. You made it so easy for us, and we are so glad we did it this." Knowing that they have preplanned leaves them feeling uplifted because they have done something for their family and it's taken care of.*

**Q. If I pay ahead, is my money safe?**

A. *Of course. This is money that they have worked hard for and saved up, and they don't want to lose it, and we don't want them to lose it. In South Carolina we have pretty strict laws about preneed planning, and it must be insured in the customer's name until the time of death. Everyone is concerned about money, and they should be. They worked hard for it. You can't lose. I laugh and tell them the only way they can lose their money is if they figure a way out of this, and if they do, please let me know!*

**Q. Me too! What information would they need to provide to you when they come for preplanning?**

A. *You would need to provide biographical information for the death certificate and obituary. We need Social Security number and a copy of the Honorable Discharge if one served in the Armed Forces.*

**Q. During the preplanning meeting(s), what types of decisions will need to be made regarding; cemetery plots, cremation vs. burial, caskets, vaults, scripture readings, music, hymn choices, pall bearers or not, eulogist? Is this done by funeral home in conjunction with clergy?**

A. *If it's a traditional ceremony (burial), you need to have selected a space at a church, synagogue or place of worship to have the ceremony and you would also need to have selected a cemetery space. Even with cremation you can bury the cremains or place them above ground in a niche. That provides a final resting place for future generations to visit. Are you on a particular budget? Most families say "We don't want to spend much money." We are always willing to abide by the family's budget. Families may provide us with any memorial requests, scripture and hymns, pall bearers and eulogist although, the clergy will go over this with them. They have to select a casket or urn and decide on services they desire. Hope this helps !!! Best Wishes !!*

Daisy, I know this information will be helpful to families who know they need to make some arrangements but are not quite sure how to proceed. Thank you very much for sharing your experience and expertise.

# Information

# 5.

## Books

A while back I was visiting my dad and was telling him a few stories about work. He looked at me and said "Son, are you writing any of this down? You have a unique perspective; you have lived through it and now you are helping families through it. You are in their homes every day!"

Now............ it's agony for me to even write a birthday card, so at first I laughed, but driving home I had a flood of ideas. I had to stop frequently to write them down. Every day, I learn something new about Alzheimer's.

There are a lot of books about AD. This is just one of many. I thought of calling this book, *"Another Alzheimer's Book,"* but I have been told several times that this one is a little different. I even have a friend who read it and calls it *"Henry's Rock-N-Roll Guide to Alzheimer's."* It kind of is. I think there is a lot of information in here that is unique because of my experiences.

Recently, I was given a book about the different activities you can do with someone who has AD. I glanced over it and here's a sample: "If your loved one likes to fish, then take him to a seafood restaurant."

Really?

How about if he likes to fish, then take him fishing?

Most books out there relate to the later stages of AD. Matter of fact, most of the information out there is related to the later stages. There isn't much information on the early-to-moderate stages and I think we are missing a real opportunity to start the care for people with dementia earlier than we do.

The one book I'm familiar with and recommend is Coach Broyles' *Playbook for Alzheimer's Caregivers*. It's the best "read" out there, and it's short for those of us who might be... *self-help book challenged*.

## The Alzheimer's Association

I hope your doctor/neurologist recommends that you go to your local Alzheimer's Association. When Mom was diagnosed our doctor didn't... or I certainly don't remember him emphasizing it if he did.

I believe just after a diagnosis is made it is in everyone's best interest for the neurologists to emphasize how important it is to find help – starting with the Alzheimer's Association. Families have their own response to AD; some families and family members will opt for denial as a coping mechanism; but for the family members who want to find activities, support groups or even participate in studies, information is vital.

Doctors play a pivotal role; they are the first, and sometimes only point of contact for families. I believe that all families should be encouraged to find support. Without guidance from the neurologists they might not ever feel connected to anything... like me. I don't remember my mom's doctors saying anything about finding help, what to do or how to proceed. I just remember "Good luck... see you in six months." I regret that I had no contact with our local Alzheimer's Association.

Here is a sample of what your local Alzheimer's Association (www.alz.org) can offer:

- Education and Training: Available for both professional care-givers and family members on a variety of topics including basics, behaviors, communication, mealtime, bathing, etc.

- Understanding the Seven Stages of Alzheimer's.

- Support Groups: Most chapters have support programs for care-givers and people with early memory loss.

- Events: Each chapter hosts a Walk to End Alzheimer's but most have other awareness and fundraising events throughout the year like golf tournaments, Dancing Stars, etc.

- Advocacy: Each chapter also hosts advocacy-related events to promote Alzheimer's awareness and needed policy changes at the legislative level.

- Trial Match: The Alzheimer's Association partners with Trial Match to help individuals find clinical trials in their area that they can participate in to further research related to dementia. Healthy individuals as well as people with dementia are needed for clinical trials.

- Helpline: Counselors are available 24/7 at 1-800-272-3900. In-person care consultations can be scheduled at your local office. Information about community resources and referrals as well as informational materials on a variety of topics are also available through the Helpline.

- Safe Return: An identification jewelry program that assists in the safe return of individuals with dementia who wander and become lost.

- Depending on what chapter is nearest you, they likely also have family events, social groups, volunteer programs and a lending library.

The Alzheimer's Association will without a doubt be your best resource to be connected. I highly recommend taking the care-giver classes. I attended these when I started Let's Go and I'm so glad I did.

### The Benefits of a Support Group

I realize support groups aren't for everyone but if you are on the fence, this email from Naomi might help you. She thought her husband Carl's condition was advancing rapidly. Carl started to refer to her as his sister. She was so hurt and became increasingly saddened by this. I could tell it was really getting to her. She then decided it was time to attend her first support group.

After a few meetings, I received this email from her.

> Hi Henry,
>
> At the Savvy Caregiver workshop, which is taught at Wesley Woods, they said to pay close attention to the emotions displayed when I am referred to by a different name. That's where my focus should be and not on the different name. If the emotions are loving then that's all that matters. It helped me tremendously!
>
> **The right information at the right time.**

When it starts to get tough, it might be a good idea for you to consider attending a class or support group. You can ask questions and listen to what others are experiencing. They have volunteers who might have personally lived through AD with a loved one and have dedicated their time in comforting people in your shoes.

I didn't make the time to attend anything when I was experiencing AD with Mom. I should have. I hope you do.

## Information OVERLOAD: My Red Book

Now I'm going to completely contradict myself. I'm pretty good at that sometimes, but what I'm after is a good balance between "knowledge is power" and going overboard with too much information and everything you "should be doing."

I have a big red binder full of information I have compiled about AD. Five years ago, I started to clip out articles and stories from the Internet, magazines and newspapers. I'd be in a doctor's office and I'd find in *People* magazine an article about Glen Campbell and his challenges, or stories about foods and nutrition, different kinds of help, and what studies were being done around the world. I found articles about choosing a day care, brochures of different businesses in the health care industry and most of all, suggestions about activities. When I would meet with the families that were interested in hiring me, I'd give them that book to have some great resources but also know I was serious.

There must be twenty new stories about Alzheimer's in the news every month. Ten are about assisted living and care choices. Two stories are about a celebrity dealing with AD. Five are about different foods and supplements that might be good for someone who has AD. A few are about a new medication, or a new procedure, or a new study...

I just have this to say...

## STOP. JUST STOP.

I remember being frustrated about all the things I was <u>supposed</u> to read and do for Mom. All the different information, in some ways, made me feel inadequate as a care-giver because it seemed to me that I was <u>supposed</u> to be doing so much more. The information was actually driving me crazy, so I say keep living the life you two enjoyed. Make a few changes gradually and take it easy on all the recommendations, **especially mine.** You are living through AD right now so you might not want to read an entire 200+ page book about it. Maybe read a little here and there. Plus, I realize the first two chapters in this book are all about things that are easier said than done. I do think though, if I had had this information when Mom was diagnosed, I would have been much better prepared as a care-giver.

Always remember – Alzheimer's is VERY DIFFICULT for everyone. I work with some families who have the means to hire all kinds of help and they can pay for the very best in care. Believe me, they are just as unhinged as the families I work with who are spending all their savings and selling their houses to afford care. Everyone is desperate and confused about what to do.

Here is the other part of Naomi's email from earlier:

> I am also attending a care-giver support group, (but I) had to skip this week due to work and I was thinking maybe I needed a break from over-focusing on Carl's condition. I know he has it but don't want to dwell on it in a negative way. Observing other people's hardship can take a toll on my energy. I may go to that one every other week. I do get good information from that group as well. I just don't want to obsess with AD and I was heading in that direction!

The best thing you can do is to simplify your life and theirs and realize what is important, how best to spend your time together, and stop worrying about how inadequate your care is. I bet you are doing a great job balancing your life and theirs.

It's an innate quality for humans (most of us) to try and constantly make things better. If you have the time and resources, try everything: supplements, a healthy diet, exercise, read about new strategies and medications. If you take care of yourself it shows. If you eat food that is good for you, you will feel better. The information in this book is to help you make a few decisions and give you a few options but what I think will make the biggest difference in YLO's life is making the time you have together count. **There is nothing more important.**

## The Age of Opinion

In this age of 24/7 fake news, I do recommend you pay attention to where the information is coming from. When you read that a doctor in France is prescribing that his patients with AD drink coconut milk (that the results are astounding), that's terrific. But maybe do a little investigating first; you might find they are selling a book...

or own a coconut farm!

Sandra, Rosebud, Poochie and
Mary Beth

# 6.

## Sisters

Mom was the oldest of four sisters: my mom Atha Alexander (Sandra), Laura (Rosebud), Evelyn (Poochie), and Mary Beth... well, she's always just been Mary Beth. Small towns and nicknames. Mom was two years older than Rosebud and they were closest in age, so they shared clothes and toys and raced for the front seat – "shot gun!" They were even married the same year.

Mom's favorite times were when we were all together as a family and traveling was a big part of that. I remember one summer when I was about ten, just about the whole family took off on a cross-country Winnebago trip out west to see Rosebud in California, and the great US of A. We went through the Arch in St. Louis, the great Corn Palace in South Dakota, Mount Rushmore, Reno, and finally our destination, San Francisco. *We were all together!* Homeward bound, we went through L.A., Arizona, the nothingness of west Texas (which I actually liked), neon Dallas, Jackson, Mississippi and finally, Wally World.

I love to travel because Mom loved to. Finding your bearings in a different place is "living." Those travel memories are without a doubt the strongest memories of my childhood. My dad took me to New York when I was eight. It was so exciting; I can just about remember every minute. I can't wait to travel with my kids and show them what I think is great.

### Don

One evening, I think the year was 1995, I got a call from Mom. "Guess who just called and I think asked me out on a date?"

"Who?" I asked. "I'll give you the initials: "D.M." Mom replied mysteriously.

Don McNeish was the dad of one of my best friends, Jim, whom I had met in the first grade. From that first date, a truly great and very special friendship evolved. Don was a true gentleman. He used to call my mom "Lady Sandra." They traveled to Europe, went on cruises and took in shows at the theater. They had many adventures together. Don made her later life very happy long after she thought these things could not happen. What a great guy!

Mom was cruising right along and was enjoying a full life. She had a second chance at romance. You couldn't have written a better story...

...and then Mom started to show signs of being a little "forgetful."

## Diagnosed

We all noticed the signs and we all ignored them. We didn't know what to do. I mean, **who does?** It was depressing to think about it. Her diagnosis was hard for me to even talk about.

Mary Beth lived just down the street from Mom and started to take action. She understood way more than I did the tasks that needed to be done. I was driving back and forth from Atlanta to Columbia, seeing Mom as much as possible, but she took the reins and drove the wagon for the first part of our journey. I am very grateful to have her for an aunt. Both Mary Beth and Poochie went all out for Mom and they included her in everything. It's wonderful being part of a very loving family. It's a blessing and one I consider to be the most important of my life.

Knowing she couldn't live up to social expectations, Mom started to withdraw a bit, but the family, along with Ardis, Kay, and a few of her other friends, kept her pretty busy. I made some difficult decisions with their help and we all worked together. With every visit, we all tried as best we could to make every moment count.

## Rosebud

Rosebud started to develop signs of dementia at about the same time as Mom. *Two of four sisters with Alzheimer's.* A few years before the diagnosis, I took a trip out to San Francisco to see Rosebud, her husband Rich, and cousins Mac and Sandie. Rosebud picked me up from the train station and we spent the whole day together. That night we three (Rosebud, Rich and I) sat down, and Rich put a glass of scotch between my fingers. For the next three hours we talked, reminisced and got to know each other. I am so glad to have had those three hours. That day was the only day I had ever had with Rosebud alone and as an adult. I learned so much about her, Mom, them growing up and of course, myself. I think about that day and how important it was to hopefully both of us. All it took was a few hours to really get to know each other because we have the same blood flowing through our hearts. We are connected by family.

Unlike my mom, Rosebud was married so she was able to stay home longer, but when Uncle Rich died in 2005, her life started to unravel. Her support at home was gone and after trying a few assisted living facilities, my cousin Mac found a residential Home for dementia for her. It's a great place and I know they are very happy with the care she is receiving. When I visited her shortly after Mom died she was doing great and still is!

Mom and Rosebud lived such different lives and had such different personalities and experiences. I have to wonder what causes Alzheimer's. Environment? Genetics? Are we predisposed to have it? Does it have something to do with the choices we make?

I talked with my uncle, Dr. Roger Sawyer, Aunt Mary Beth's husband; he is a biology professor at the University of South Carolina, the finest University in the world. Roger reminds me of and exemplifies the best qualities of Doc from Steinbeck's *Cannery Row*.

I asked him how he felt genetics impacted the predisposition to Alzheimer's.

> *(Roger) Dr. Lah has provided a very realistic view of Alzheimer's, as I understand the studies I have read. The interactions between one's genetic composition and life-style choices are complicated, and it is clear that there are no definitive answers for either disease (AD and dementia) at this time, but a number of avenues are being explored. Although my research interests are in the area of evolutionary genetics, I do follow reports on Alzheimer's since Mary Beth's sisters Rosebud and your mother, Sandra, came down with the disease at an early age.*

> *An article in the New England Journal of Medicine in 2012 by Bateman and his colleagues (Clinical and Biomarker Changes in Dominantly Inherited Alzheimer's Disease; N. Engl. J. Med. 367: 795-804) is of interest. This rare form of inherited Alzheimer's disease (accounts for only ~1% of cases) is being used to identify biological changes that precede the disease, years or even decades before symptoms of the disease appear. For example, changes in brain chemistry have been detected 15 years before expected symptom*

*onset. This same article points out that mutations in one of three genes have been identified that cause alterations in brain chemistry.*

*The answer to your question about genetics is yes, there are genetic components of Alzheimer's that are being studied. A major international partnership known as DIAN (Dominantly Inherited Alzheimer's Network) has been established and is seeking ways to use pre-symptomatic biomarkers to eventually prevent and treat the disease. Since this form of Alzheimer's makes up only ~1% of the cases, there are clearly other environmental and genetic factors involved.*

Thanks Roger. It's great to have someone with your background who can keep us up to date and informed. You and Uncle Gary are the best brothers-in-law Mom could have ever had.

## Sandra's Oral History

Ardis and Kay were Mom's best friends. Mom worked together with Ardis at the university. When Mom faced retiring earlier than she would have liked because of her symptoms with AD, Ardis took it upon herself to help Mom write a book. (She knew how important her family was and her natural interest in her own family background). She would visit with Mom and go over the family history and would ask Mom to explain pictures of her growing up, my childhood, vacations, and trips. They would talk for hours about Mom's life and Ardis wrote it all down, for me. It was a gift to me from Mom for Christmas in 2004. That book is the most important possession I own.

My mom came from a huge family. Her grandmother was one of sixteen! Mom always had great stories about her growing up in Pageland and Lancaster, South Carolina, with her extended family. Some of them were real characters! Unlike today, most of the kids didn't move away so there were great uncles, aunts and cousins all over the county. Forty years ago, we would have 300 to 400 people at our family reunions. Mom kept in touch with almost all of them. It was very important to her to know her family and her roots.

Here is an excerpt from "The Book":

*Then there was the time during my sophomore year in high school in Coral Gables when I went to lunch with Gary Cooper. That spring, a boy at the local military academy and two of his buddies invited*

*me and two of my girlfriends to a dance at the academy. Well, it just
so happened that my date was the brother of Patricia O'Neal, and
she and Gary Cooper had been "an item" (as they used to say) for a
number of years. Gary Cooper was in town doing something with a
movie and Patricia was with him. The day before the dance, Patricia
O'Neal and Gary Cooper invited the three couples to have lunch with
them at their hotel. I remember people coming to the table to get
Gary Cooper's autograph. Everyone in the dining room was looking
in our direction and whispering, and there I was sitting right next to
him. I was absolutely giddy. He was very nice and polite to the three
of us. He wore casual clothes and no cowboy hat! We didn't have a
camera, so there never was a picture of us with him. Mama was so
disappointed she never got to see him, and was heard to say "What
a waste" about the whole episode. "I'm sure they giggled through
the entire lunch!"*

### An interview with Ardis

The writing of "Sandra's Oral History."

Hello Ardis,

I can't thank you enough for this book. Every now and then I pull "The
Book" out and re-read it. I get to re-live some great memories. I know this
book will help me introduce my kids to their grandmother, something very
important to me.

Q. **Where did you get the idea to write a book about my
mother's life?**

A. *As your mother's Alzheimer's disease progressed, she was no longer
able to shop or do errands on her own, so I would go with her. Each
time I arrived at her house I found her surrounded by photographs
and clippings she had collected over the years, some of them dating
back to her great grandparents. She knew she had Alzheimer's,
and she knew she would lose her memory. I realized she needed
someone to talk to about her pictures and about what she did
remember. One of her greatest worries was that soon she would no
longer be able to share those memories with you or her sisters, all of
whom were younger than she. I asked her if she liked the idea of the
two of us working together to write a short memory for
each picture.*

*I wouldn't call it a book, although it surely did become a history of your mother's life in her own words. Rather, it is more of a scrapbook of her pictures and clippings with a brief narrative beside each one. That was important to her. She wanted the original photographs coupled with her memories to pass on to you.*

**Q. Did you have any formal outline, or was it spontaneous?**

A. *I had no outline. Your mother was remembering her life... it was her decision about what would be covered in the telling of it. If we hadn't used the random selection of pictures that interested her, I guess we might have needed an outline of some kind.*

**Q. What was the process you used?**

A. *Your mother was no longer able to think about her life in terms of a progressive time line. The project was never approached as an oral history. Instead, we sat in my study with boxes of photos on the floor, your mother relaxed and comfortable on the sofa with a Coke and some cookies. I would say, "Sandra, pull out one of your pictures and tell me about it." While she talked, I sat at my computer typing her response. This worked much better than taking a video of her. She could relax and take her time. She didn't feel as if she had to be performing for the camera, and, in this case, it became a joke between the two of us because for fifteen years she had typed what I had dictated, and now the tables were turned. She liked that!*

*Each time she talked about an item, I placed a number on it, and then I placed the same number on the typed comments. We would spend about two hours each time we met, or until I sensed she was tiring. After about three months we had assembled nearly seventy of her favorite photos and clippings, but nothing was in chronological order. I cut and clipped all of the typed memories to each of the photos with a matching number. I then spread every item out on the floor and kept moving them around until they fell into a time line. Finally they were arranged in a bound picture album (each page with a glassine cover).*

*For the two genealogies of your mother's family going back ten (1700) and twelve (1619) generations, I used one of many on-line resources. She loved talking about our family history.*

**Q. Was she at all apprehensive trying to remember?**

A. *Not at all. I think, in large part, it was because she was under no pressure. She didn't have to try to fit her memories into a timeline, and, therefore, never had the feeling of "I can't remember what happened next." Since we were about the same age, I would often share some of my own experiences (wedding, children at a certain age, fashions of the day, celebration of holidays, college life, etc.), and that would trigger a host of other memories for her. And, she felt the whole idea was HER project. She was putting together a Christmas present for you. She was in charge. She selected the pictures, and when we were done I sat down with her and we read the entire book together with the understanding that everything had to be done to her liking or it would be changed (nothing was!). I think that was important.*

**Q. If someone were beginning a project like this, what tips could you pass on?**

A. *I'm certainly no expert on oral histories. This is the only one I have ever done. Maybe the only tip I have is let the process be fun, like two old friends sitting together and remembering "the good old days." As much as possible, make it their project, not yours, go with the flow, and it will become an accomplishment of which they are proud, and that is important.*

Thanks Ardis. These are perfect. I think what you have offered because of her will be a great help to many more.

**Thank you for everything you did for Mom.**

# Intermission

# 7.

*Brazil* was one of Mom's favorite movies, Terry Gilliam's insane movie about a bureaucratic future gone very wrong.

My Mom was just "that cool."

She loved going to the movies. They were a big part of her life. She always had a standing date on the weekend with a few of her friends to see a movie and she wasn't afraid to experiment. It didn't matter if it was Hollywood, Indie, or foreign, she appreciated the medium. We had a great independent movie theater in Columbia called The Nickelodeon; a small, old-fashioned movie house right behind the state capital building. Growing up, I saw a lot of movies there that shaped my life. I also saw a bunch of bad ones there too, but that's part of the deal.

Mom appreciated the talent in writing, directing, and acting. She valued the thoughtfulness of the art, and most of all she appreciated good storytelling.

I took her to see movies up until the very end, even when she wasn't talking anymore. I'd pick out a movie that I knew she would like. We would get popcorn and watch the trailers. I knew she was enjoying it. I could just tell. She was living in the present and giving it her best to muster all her concentration. She would reach for the popcorn and give me a small smile. Nick Cage or Parker Posey walking through Washington Square. A few kids standing under the Eiffel Tower with accordion music. Maybe a period piece with great costumes and a big social dance... on a 30-foot screen! Who wouldn't enjoy that?!

Her favorites were Gary Cooper – because, of course, they had lunch together! Then there was Paul Newman, and Bill Forsyth's *That Sinking Feeling* and *Local Hero* – we must have listened to that soundtrack a thousand times. One time I remember she told me, under her breath, and with no one in earshot, "I loved *Pulp Fiction*."

111

The movies were special for both of us. Here is a letter I wrote to actor John Cusack after watching one of his movies.

————

Summer 2005

Hey John,

My name is Henry Watts. I'm writing from Atlanta Georgia. I take my mom to see a movie every other weekend. Last week we saw *Must Love Dogs*. We both loved it. I too have watched *Dr. Zhivago* twenty times. I have loved Julie Christie ever since I saw *Darling.*

Your characters and your movies have always been like a thread of the fabric woven between myself and my mom, probably not unlike a lot of 38-year-olds. She (along with a few ex-girlfriends) have sometimes compared me to you.

My mom has Alzheimer's now. She was diagnosed about five years ago. She is fading. I can't tell you how important it is to make that mental contact (which happens less and less with every visit), but for one minute after we saw your movie, I had her back.

As we walked out of the theater she said, *"I loved the movie! I loved the characters! And I love that John Cusack!"*

I don't know if you know anybody who has Alzheimer's but it is a real battle to remember anybody's first name much less their last name. We made contact. Me, you, and Mom. Your movie brought the old Mom back for a brief moment, something I'll never forget. We talked about it for the rest of the day. Actually, I talked about it for the rest of the day. She nodded and said "yes" a lot, smiled, and slowly drifted back into her own world.

I just wanted to let you know you were there when I was a teenager and you are there for me now. I appreciate your work.

Thanks John.

Your Pal,

Henry

# Understanding Limitations

# 8.

**Just Holding On**

Even though the symptoms of AD, in most cases, come on gradually you would think that you would get to know the disease, understand each stage and be ready for the next; but somehow AD just doesn't work that way. At least it didn't for me nor has it worked that way for my client's families. One day you are on top of the situation and everything is "under control", but Alzheimer's has a way of morphing itself into several different challenges at once. This is how you can gradually lose control.

In the early stages of the disease the choices you make can affect the quality of life for both you and the person you are caring for. In the later stages your choices can be limited for a number of reasons. One being that the dementia has taken away their motivation and now they might not be interested in doing much of anything. This lack of interest could be caused by a number of reasons: YLO might be intimidated in carrying on a conversation and embarrassed by what they can't comprehend any more. It might be the uncertainty of leaving home or even coordination issues (afraid of falling). This withdrawal might be their way of stepping back from the confusion. What is important for them now is trying to hold on to a few things they find comforting and familiar – repetitive behavior, asking the same questions, reading the same letters, sleeping all day, cleaning, organizing and in general, searching for ways to keep themselves grounded.

This can be very confusing to a care-giver because you might think "A visit with the grandkids or being around friends is just what Mom needs" but because everything has become confusing to them, it might be that the only way to lessen their anxiety is just by doing... nothing. This is the burden of Alzheimer's. Sometimes the best thing you can do to help YLO is to hold their hand, reassure and tell them that everything is OK and let them do whatever they need to "get by." AD is a great challenge because at times it can deprive you, the care-giver, of being able to comfort YLO.

Alzheimer's can and will change how you spend time with YLO so don't feel guilty about not taking Pop to the baseball games anymore. Realizing that those days are over is one of the saddest parts of AD, but moving forward and understanding what YLO would prefer to do will help you be a better care-giver.

## A Very Special Relationship

What I have observed in the last eight years is, in most cases, care-giving for a spouse is extremely more difficult and intense than care-giving for a parent. If your husband or your wife has AD, I can't imagine what you are going through right now. You chose each other. You live in the same home, eat breakfast and dinner together, go on trips together, have the same friends, and live the same life. Being married allows you to take on the world – together. Now, AD has tipped the balance you two have shared for so long and sadly, you are gradually losing support from your life-partner.

I wanted to address this because I have been to too many meetings, classes, support groups, and conferences where I have heard someone say to a spouse who is care-giving for their husband or wife, "I know what you are going through, my parent has dementia."

Honestly, we have no idea what they are going through.

When?

# 9.

## An Interview with Kara Johnson

This is an interview with Kara Johnson, a care consultant at the Alzheimer's Association in Atlanta. I have asked her a few questions about "When?" Timing can be so difficult – when does someone need to see a neurologist? When might someone start to consider in-home care or assisted living for their loved one? If you need to ask someone who helps people with the hard questions, Kara is the best. She has been a great resource for me and has helped me be better at what I do. I value her friendship.

**Bio**: Kara earned her MSW from UNC-Chapel Hill with a concentration on Aging/Gerontology. She has worked in the field of aging for seven years, having served as the director of an adult day center for adults with dementia and related disorders as well as the social services director of a continuing care retirement community.

Hello Kara,

Thank you for talking with me today. I have a few questions about some important decisions that families might have to make.

> **Q.** **(Henry) When do you go to the doctor/neurologist because you might think YLO has dementia?**
>
> A. *(Kara) Now. Getting an accurate diagnosis will lead to accurate and, hopefully, effective treatment options. There are temporary/ reversible causes of memory loss including some types of infections, thyroid disorders and as a side effect to some medications. You'll want to immediately rule out (or treat) any reversible cause of memory loss. If the diagnosis is dementia, you'll want to find out what type of dementia. There are over 90 different types of dementia and not all dementias are treated the same way. Finding*

*the best treatment options for your loved one as early on as possible will increase the potential efficacy of those options.*

**Q. When do you tell friends and family about an Alzheimer's diagnosis?**

A. *I think this depends on a number of things. What stage is the person with the diagnosis in? How do they feel about their diagnosis? Perhaps they are still very high-functioning and not ready for the stigma that can be attached to such a diagnosis. The sad truth is that you and your loved one may lose some friends after a diagnosis becomes public. Some people just do not understand or know how to be supportive of someone with a diagnosis of dementia. It's not okay but it is something to be prepared for and to talk about as a family. There is also the possibility that the person with the diagnosis will never be able to accept that as their reality because they have progressed beyond being able to recognize their limitations. In this case, the family/primary care-giver will want to consider reaching out to their support networks (and widening them if possible) early so that others can be attuned to the fact that they will need assistance and support.*

**Q. When do you see a financial adviser/elder law attorney?**

A. *Absolutely as soon as possible. First of all, if the person with dementia is in the very early stages, it is best to involve them in the decision-making process so that they can sign forms identifying a Power of Attorney, etc. if possible. You will also want as much time as possible to plan for the future financially. If veteran's or government benefits are needed, the earlier you can have an elder law attorney look at your assets/finances, the better.*

**Q. When is it time to stop traveling?**

A. *A person does not have to stop traveling and attending social events because of a diagnosis of dementia, but there are some things you should try to be prepared for. Early on in the disease process a person with dementia may be more "clingy" to a spouse or loved one in social situations because they are afraid of making a mistake socially and so they may rely heavily on others to correct/fill in gaps for them. Understanding this as the care-giver will help you to be more empathetic and patient with the person with dementia in such situations.*

*As far as traveling, many of us have probably experienced the brief disorientation that comes with waking up in a hotel room when traveling and having to think "now where am I again?" A person with memory loss may feel this way often or for longer. You'll want to be ready to remind and reassure them of where they are and where you're going/why. Be sure to pack your patience as well as your sense of humor and adventure! You'll also want to be sure to pack things that make the person with dementia feel the most comfortable/relaxed – favorite clothes, relaxing music for car rides and any other favorite items that may be comforting. Be ready to take breaks from traveling and activities so that the person with dementia can "re-charge" as/if needed.*

**Q. When is it time to consider adult day care? I love what they offer. It's a great option for those who fit.**

A. *I think there are actually many reasons why someone might choose an adult day care for their loved one but then, I am a BIG proponent of adult day centers. They do provide a safe place for the person with dementia as well as respite for care-givers, but they have many other benefits as well: A sense of purpose – we are all searching for a sense of purpose in our daily lives and that is something – that does not change when a person gets dementia. Have they always been doers? Fixers? Helpers? Creators? Listeners? Sharers? How can their activity needs best be met? This is one of the jobs of the staff at an adult day center to discover. We also all benefit from socialization and stimulation. Benefits may include improved mood, better sleep/ wake cycles, more alertness and a decrease in agitation. Most adult day centers incorporate some type of physical exercise into their programs as well, which is invaluable as a mental, emotional and physical health benefit. Then there's a sense of belonging that many individuals feel at an adult day center. This can translate into a positive emotional memory of the center and its staff/participants. There is usually an adjustment period, as Henry alluded to and adult day centers are not for everyone. However, I have seen some of the most opposed people thrive in the day center environment so don't give up too early! You may even consider hiring a companion to go with the person in the beginning so that they get a lot of one-on-one attention until they feel more comfortable with the program/environment.*

**Q.  What are your thoughts on having your parent move closer to you?**

A.  *There is MUCH to consider before making the decision to move a loved one closer to or in with you. Where will you and the person with dementia have the most support systems? Which area has better resources, i.e., specialists, facilities if needed in the future, senior centers/programming, Medicare/Medicaid resources, etc. How will other family members be impacted by such a move? If you are trying to develop a good plan and you and your loved one are in separate states, several good first steps would be to call the Alzheimer's Association in both areas so you can compare resources available in both states and then to consider hiring a Geriatric Care Manager(GCM). A GCM is a professional, usually a licensed social worker, who can come in and make a full assessment of the person with dementia including safety concerns and health needs and can then help you and other family members develop a care plan based on that assessment. Having an unbiased third-party professional step in can be an invaluable tool if there are a lot of "cooks in the kitchen" who need to get on the same page OR if you are the only responsible party and you are miles and miles away from the person with dementia.*

**Q.  When is it time to hire in-home care?**

A.  *In-home care is a great tool that can help people stay in their home for as long as possible, which is what most people desire. Maybe they just need someone to do medication reminders, light housekeeping, meal prep, errands, but otherwise can manage their activities of daily living (ADLs) independently. Or maybe they just need help getting started in the morning but then they're good to go for the rest of the day. In-home care is usually pretty expensive whether you are hiring a companion (usually an untrained professional who manages household tasks or provides companionship) or a certified nursing assistant (CNA – a licensed professional who can help with ADL's including but not limited to bathing, dressing, toileting, feeding and transfers). You will want to be a good steward of your loved one's financial resources and if you're hiring someone to provide between 12-24 hour care a day in the home, you're usually spending a pretty good bit. If finances are not a concern, that's wonderful. If they are, you may want to consider either pairing in-home care with adult day center supervision or the possibility that it is time for your loved one to move into a facility where they will have the 24-hour supervision that is needed to keep them safe.*

**Q. When is it time for assisted living?**

A. *Again, this is not a one-size-fits-all answer. Some families naturally come to the conclusion that assisted living facility (ALF) placement is needed when their loved one needs 24-hour supervision that cannot adequately be provided at home. Others come to this conclusion when the type of care needed exceeds what they are physically able to do at home (for example, maybe the person wanders constantly or needs increased physical assistance with ADLs that the primary care-giver is not able to provide safely). Still others realize that the best way to preserve their own mental and physical health as a spouse/child/care-giver is to spend their energy making each visit special as opposed to just surviving each day. Still others may find that the person with dementia just LOVES being around other people all the time and sees that a memory care unit chocked full of activities all day long and into the evenings is just what they need/ want to keep them as happy as possible. There are a million ways that people may begin to ask themselves the question, "Is it time for a move?" The best advice I have to offer is to talk to one of the counselors at the Alzheimer's Association. They will be able to help you sort out the practical questions (How much will it cost? What should I look for in a facility? Do you have a list of places near me? ), as well as help you sort through the emotional weight of a decision like this.*

**Q. When is it time for a nursing home (skilled care facility)?**

A. *Similar to the last answer, there are many reasons why someone may find themselves considering a nursing home (NH) or skilled nursing facility (SNF) (these are interchangeable terms) for their loved one. In Georgia, our new ALF regulations were recently adjusted to help people be able to age in place longer in assisted living settings. It used to be that as a resident's physical needs increased, the ALF would have to move the person out, usually recommending nursing home care. The new regulations still require that residents be at a certain level when they enter the ALF, but allow residents to age in place longer through facility-regulated supportive care/services, like hospice and other medical provisions. That said, there is still sometimes the need, for medical reasons, to move to a care setting that has a higher staff to patient ratio or has more RN/physician coverage than an ALF may have. Other reasons a nursing home might be a more appropriate placement would include financial (Medicaid helps cover the cost of nursing home care in Georgia, but not ALF care), proximity to family or quality of care.*

**Q.  When is it time for you to realize that you are only human?**

A.  *It is never too early to realize that you are only human, that you are only one person and that you cannot do it all on your own. Think about all of the jobs you are likely trying to do yourself: Accountant, driver, nursing assistant, housekeeper, launderer, activity coordinator, appointment scheduler, cook, and so on. Not to mention you're other role(s) as spouse/daughter/son/friend, etc. Who has time to be anything but stressed when you're trying to do the work of a whole team of people all the time! Rarely can all of this be conquered by one person alone. It takes a team of supporters to care for a person with dementia. We recommend that you start expanding your support networks as soon as you can: church, support groups, the Alzheimer's Association, friends you can rely on, family who can lend a hand or an ear, physicians who are familiar with dementia and will make time to listen when there are concerns. Make time for yourself when possible. More specifically, plan time for yourself into the weekly schedule. Reach out to your support network regularly to ask for advice or assistance, take a break, find time to laugh, etc. Care-giving is an enormous job and it is not an easy one. Take care of yourself so you can take care of the person that you love.*

Thanks Kara. These are all terrific!

I told Kara that these answers were so good that I needed to change some of my writing in the book. I started thinking in a more informed way. These really are great.

# A Progression of Care

# 10.

Caring for someone who has AD is not the same as caring for a healthy aging parent or spouse. If YLO seems to be confused with a few simple tasks, or is slowly withdrawing, it's not because they are getting older. Alzheimer's is a disease. As this disease progresses, it can be very difficult to care for someone, especially in the later stages. Since in-home care and assisted living can be such a big part of caring for someone who has AD, I have divided this chapter into four parts.

In Part 1, *In-Home Care and Adult Day Care*. Here is where I think caring for someone is the most complex and confusing for families: the in-between period, also known as "Stage 4, moderate cognitive decline." Twenty-four-hour care is not needed, but maybe four to eight hours a day is. I start with two options for YLO, "in-home care" and "adult day care." They both can be tremendous assets in helping you care for YLO. I also have a few suggestions on how adult day care could be a little more assessable.

In Part 2, *Assisted Living*, I'll cover assisted living from the point of view, including memory care and skilled care. I'll offer suggestions on choosing the right facility and moving YLO in. I'll also cover what a short stay in a hospital might be like and what you might expect in a rehab/physical therapy facility.

In Part 3, *A Few Minor Adjustments*, I'll offer some recommendations and suggestions to the facilities themselves to make assisted living a better experience for residents. I think a few simple, inexpensive remedies could make assisted living more attractive for all of us.

In Part 4, *Why I Really like Assisted Living* is a story about "Pat", Mom's best friend at the Lowman Home and why the benefits and social aspects of assisted living are so important to me.

> **Here are a few care options for when the task becomes too difficult for you and your family to maintain quality of care.**

# Part 1.

# In-Home Care and Adult Day Care.

### In-Home Care

Everyone would like to live at home as long as possible. The thought of moving into assisted living to most people is beyond frightening.

"You are going to put me in a nursing home!?"

"Why?"

"In-Home Care", "Companion Care", or "Personal Care" is care in your own home. This type of care can either assist you in some of your caregiving duties or take over most of them. You can have someone come over a few hours a week to give you a break or around-the-clock care when it is time for the difficult challenge of the later stages of AD. Sometimes, these in-home care-givers are called CNA's (Certified Nursing Assistants), sitters or companions. Sometimes they are called caretakers. I'm not sure why. They *give* care. Plus – it sounds like someone taking care of a barn.

I am a companion. I am usually involved in the earlier stages and help families with all the transitions to the later stages and in most cases until the very end. The right person will enable YLO to stay at home a lot longer. I work hard in keeping people active and believe that can make a huge difference in delaying the very expensive types of care.

Some companies offer an option where a registered nurse can stop by and supervise care. Usually an evaluation will take place and then they will make recommendations based on what your needs are and what type of care YLO might need. The Alzheimer's Association has a list of care-givers in your area. Senior centers are also a great place to find information about in-home care. There are lots to choose from: national chains, locally owned businesses, or individuals.

### Finding the Right Person

A family I was working with hired some extra help. The new care-giver was happy to be there at first but shortly after her arrival, I could tell things were not playing out as she anticipated. It was a difficult situation and she just wasn't up to the task. Of course my client reciprocated her attitude by becoming even more difficult, so I suggested a new hire. The new care-giver had the right personality and was a much better fit.

## Radioactive

If healthy living is one of your concerns (it would be for me), then it might be important to choose someone who looks like they take care of themselves.

## Adult Day Care

If YLO needs supervision throughout the day, adult day care is a great option. (Rewind back to Pg. 121.) I completely agree with Kara on all counts. A few years ago, I was a bit cold towards a few adult day care centers, but hearing and witnessing many success stories, I now understand that these places really are great **for those who fit**.

My favorite by far is one I visited that two guys ran in the back of a church. They had maybe twelve people with varying degrees of dementia, a few people in wheelchairs. The guys brought in good homemade food. They were playing dominoes and *most everyone* was participating and actually having a good time. Those who were there, their spouses, and their children, didn't have to worry during that time. That is worth gold.

I have a client who just started going to one. He is a retired colonel so his benefits through VA are paying for it. He loves it and looks forward to going. Six months ago, a team of wild horses couldn't have dragged him through the front door.

If you have tried it and it didn't go well, wait three or four months and try again. If it's a success and it works, you won't believe how much better both of your lives will be. You will know YLO will be having a good day and you will get a much deserved and needed break.

> Before you visit a day care facility you do need to prepare yourself – walking into one for the first time is going to be difficult. That might be your first introduction to seeing other people who are a little farther along than YLO is. It's like walking into a nursing home for the first time. They are both worlds we are never ready for, but they are certainly reminders of what is really going on.

## My Experience

My work has taken me to several adult day cares or day-care programs in Atlanta and what I have finally conceded about adult day care is that it's not for everyone. *But what is?* I don't want to be unfair to adult day care.

They try hard to get it right and some of them really are great. If you give it some time and stay committed for it to work, most people in adult day care will thrive, as Kara said. I have walked into a few where almost everyone there was involved, socializing, laughing, and enjoying the day so I DO NOT want to discourage you from considering adult day care.

I have really struggled writing this part of the book because like I said, I do not want to discourage you from trying something that could be so beneficial to YLO, but I also need to be honest about what my experience has been.

## A Very Solvable Problem

I have spent a good part of my time on this planet with people who have AD. I'm not in "the system" at all and I answer to no one except the families I work with. I believe I'm in a good place to appreciate what people are trying to do with dementia... and I certainly have my opinions of where they fall short. I am continuously astounded by our healthcare system regarding dementia care and its complete lack of understanding of what families are going through.

I have plenty more "opinions" about changes that need to be made in the last chapter of the book. I also have a much more involved and current list of problems with solutions (updated every month) in my Let's Go newsletter. Go to www.AtlantaLetsGo.com and click on *Newsletter*. You can help with your own suggestions and together we can solve these problems.

Here is what I perceive is "the problem" with adult day care: Groupings. Why do we put people who have become forgetful with people in wheelchairs, or advanced stage AD or Down syndrome? That makes no sense to me. What activity can they all participate in? None. The groupings should be considered on cognitive abilities, similar interests, and similar personalities. By targeting people experiencing the same difficulties with their disease, adult day care could offer a much higher level of activity and freedom.

Here is an email from Shelly. I was trying to help Shelly place Scott into day care and it was just not going to work.

> *Even though Scott cannot do many of the normal day-to-day things, he believes that he can. This is where I think we need to adjust our thinking. He would never play bingo when he was cognitively well, let alone now that he is not. Scott knows that he is in day care but*

*he does not understand what he is doing there. He is furious and we both know that his dementia is fairly advanced and he needs to be there. Most of the people there can't really do anything for themselves, yet I believe if he were assigned some duties that he could be reasonably successful with, he would be happier. He can set the table, clear the table, wipe off tables, carry plates, help the older ladies into chairs, etc. I think all the things they are trying to do now can be done from a different angle without making the folks wonder what the heck they are doing there. Do dog therapy. Do something similar to Arts for Alzheimer's. Bring in a good movie. Pop some popcorn. Make it fun. Have a cookout! But make it feel like they are at a social event instead of at "day care."*

This email is a good example of why it has been difficult placing some of my clients into adult day care. Quite honestly, if I had AD and had to cut out a picture of a duck or heard "B-19... Bingo!" I might be headed for the exits too.

I think "groupings" are a solvable problem and could help those who might be a little more apprehensive toward adult day care. Today in some cities, there are a few AD specific memory day cares, so the world of one-size fits all is slowly changing. I have an idea for adult day care for men. It's called The Lodge. (www.TheLodgeAtlanta.org)

# Part 2.

# Assisted Living Facilities

I have heard this. Maybe you have too.

> *"I promised Dad I would never put him away in some nursing home! I'm not going to abandon him. He took care of me and I'll do the same for him."*

These might even be your thoughts. Seems very reasonable to me. When I was considering moving Mom into a Home and was having doubts and feeling guilty, one of her friends told me, "You know, Henry, your mom isn't just getting older, she is sick. She has Alzheimer's. Sick people, who have the resources, are institutionalized. It's the most humane thing to do."

A fairly stark interpretation, but it was something I needed to hear. Agree or not, I completely understand if you are not going to take Dad down to the "Home" and put him away. These next pages are all about assisted living so they might not be for you.

I'll make no bones about it: I am a big fan of assisted living. It is a last resort, but to many families, a very necessary one. I placed my own mother in one. I have helped sons and daughters place their parents in assisted living and I have helped husbands and wives (a crushing decision) place their spouses in these facilities. In doing this, I have seen what seemed like a hopeless situation turn into something hopeful through assisted living.

---

**You have done everything possible to keep YLO at home.
Now it's time to consider assisted living.**

---

### An End and a Beginning

> *"You Can't Always Get What You Want"*
>
> *The Rolling Stones* [1]

Many of us have memories of walking into a nursing home as a kid. I think it's a worldwide known fact that nursing homes are not where you want to be – a bad experience with a great aunt in a nursing home or seeing a movie where someone is living in one of the terrible ones. Nursing homes get a bad rap, and some deserve it. Even today, with all the regulations,

132

some are still really bad. I completely understand why some people just can't accept putting their husband or mom in a "Home." Whatever the reason, I'm sure everyone would rather stay in his or her home. That's a given, but I believe an understanding of the different levels of care and the different kinds of homes will advance the cause for assisted living. A nursing home is an assisted living facility, but it's a very advanced stage facility for people who can't do much for themselves. Today, nursing homes are called "skilled care facilities." When you are looking for a Home for Dad and he has early signs of AD, you might be looking for a retirement community, not a nursing home. There is a big difference between an assisted living home, a memory care facility, and a skilled care or nursing home. I was never quite sure of the differences until I started looking for Mom.

## Definitions and Differences

I asked my friend Darby to help us out with the definitions and differences of assisted living. She is the only person I have met along my caregiving adventure with whom I have had a conversation about Ziggy Stardust! Darby has become a good friend in this world of care. I have been to a lot of assisted living facilities. I have my problems with some of them, but I know wherever Darby is, those people are going to get the very best care. I mean that. I'm not saying that because she is my pal. I'm saying that because it's true. I trust her. If I end up in one, I hope she is there.

**Bio**: Darby Dreger Tracey, CTRS (Certified Therapeutic Recreation Specialist), Community Relations Director, Dogwood Forest of Dunwoody Assisted Living and Memory Care

Hello Darby,

### Q.  Could you give us a quick definition of each of these?

- *Retirement community: (Darby) A place that usually has an age requirement of 55 and over. Typically, they are apartments or cottages, and do not provide any direct care or services.*

- *In-home care or companion care: This is a broad area, but it could include: light housekeeping, meal preparation, errands, incidental transportation, grocery shopping and recreational activities or personal care for bathing, grooming, hygiene, transferring, toileting and other needs.*

- *Assisted living facilities: Assisted living is designed to provide residents with assistance in basic activities of daily living, such as bathing, grooming, dressing, and toileting needs. Medication management and reminders are oftentimes available in certain states. Some states will allow skilled setting to manage medications. Residents in assisted living can be as independent as they can, and often become more independent because of the support services provided. Along with the care, assisted living communities offer many amenities, such as three meals a day served in a dining room, a full activity program with a bus for outings, transportation to doctors, housekeeping and laundry, on-site therapy, and nicely appointed common area spaces.*

- *Assisted living homes/houses: Residential homes converted into assisted living facilities. They are usually smaller communities with more personalized care.*

- Memory care: *(More on page 156) In most cases, memory care units are available within an assisted living community. Memory care specializes in providing care and services to those residents who have progressed Alzheimer's disease, dementia, Parkinson's disease, and other memory deficits. Typically, the memory care area is a secured living space, with a secured area for outdoor patio access and walking space. The memory care staff are specially trained to assist people with dementia and impaired cognition, and the activity programming is designed for residents with Alzheimer's and dementia.*

- *Skilled care facility/nursing: These are facilities that are designed to provide long-term nursing care, and rehabilitation, as well as other skilled services. In these facilities, the residents are under the care of a physician, and a physician will be available for emergencies. These facilities will have licensed nursing professionals, and other support services, such as social workers and therapists.*

- *Hospice care: This is care designed to give supportive care to those who are in the final stages of a terminal illness. The goal with this care is to focus on quality of life and comfort measures (palliative care), rather than a cure involving aggressive treatment. Hospice care is designed to enable residents to live free of pain, and to live each remaining day in comfort. Hospice care can be provided in the patient's home, an assisted living community, nursing home, or hospital setting.*

- *Age in place: At this time, the definitions for this can be all over the place. I basically try to keep it simple. Aging in place is the ability to be able to live in one's own home, or chosen environment, for as long as one wants to regardless of age, ability or illness.*

Darby will be back later for an interview. (Pg.139)

Assisted living is an umbrella term and can be used to describe a rehab center or memory care community etc. The differences in the various sub categories can be subtle; you can go to a rehab center and just down the hall (or next door, or your roommate!) is the nursing wing. Also, in Georgia we have what is called "Personal Care Communities." These can be a great option for those with early to moderate memory loss. Because the residents are able to complete certain tasks and maintain a level of personal care for themselves, these communities can offer extensive activities and outings. It's not a facility where you can age in place because when some one has reached a certain point, the staff usually uses a scale to describe a level of care that is needed, the resident will have to move into memory or nursing care.

**The Decision**

If you are looking for an assisted living facility/senior living community let me just say, *"Good for you!"* Most people don't want you to feel obligated to take care of their every need. My mom sure didn't and I wouldn't either. She said a number of times, "I did not raise you to look after me. You live your life." The last thing in the world I would want if I had AD is for James and Dylan, my children, to put me up in a room in their home if they have children of their own, especially if I'm not good company. But that's me. My thoughts may be different from yours. I grew up an only child. Mom was a very private person, and the mother/son dynamic is very different to that of the mother/daughter relationship. It would not have worked on a number of levels. I know a lot of families do this and it works great or it works because it has to. Don't get me wrong here. If you are able to care for a parent who has dementia by allowing them to move in, that's terrific.

A personal note to my family:

> *Darcy, James and Dylan – If, for any reason, I should need a lot of care, and if we have the resources, this would be my request:*

*"Please, put me in a Home. You live your life! **I trust you and you should trust yourself.** I know you would open your own home to me, but I have a disease. Caring for me is going to be so much more difficult than caring for mentally healthy Dad. Send me some grandchildren art to put on my mini-fridge and come and visit when you can. It will make me happy to know you are happy!"*

If it were possible to have sixty seconds of absolute clarity with YLO, I bet he or she would use it to try and tell you, "I want what is best for you! Stop with all this. I'm driving you crazy, but I can't help it, so please move me into assisted living."

If you are having doubts (because I know you are), look back ten years ago when YLO was of sound mind and body. Would he or she have said, "I do not want to be a burden to you. I'll be the first in line." They would know you are raising your own children or putting fifty hours a week at the office. Now they might sing a different tune because they think you are abandoning them. Well, you know who's changed their minds? No one. Their mind actually hasn't changed – *it's the Alzheimer's talking.* Don't listen. Keep with the original plan. It's what YLO wanted and it's what you agreed to. The hard part about AD is not taking everything personally. Don't forget that it's the disease, not them and **not you.**

### A Plan

When the symptoms of AD overtake your lives completely, you might be exhausted from so many restless nights and so many battles with YLO. They might take all of their frustration out on you so you might not be at your best at making decisions. This is the time when you look back and thank yourself for coming up with a plan and when taking advice from friends and professionals really counts.

### The Plan:

1. Set up a budget for an assisted living facility.

2. Investigate your options. **Are you looking for assisted living or memory care?** Check out some in the neighborhood or other convenient areas.

3. Talk with the staff. Get a feel for each facility.

4. Investigate all the necessary steps for a controlled move.

Yes, it's depressing to think about all this. It is a very difficult step. Acknowledging the problem and reviewing your options will help you in the long run... and it can be a long run.

> Not acknowledging what is happening is in itself a way to deal and cope. Personally, after caring for someone who had AD and now seeing others do the same, I don't think it's the best "way."

## Why a Move Might be Necessary

When deciding whether assisted living/memory care is appropriate, there are many considerations that you need to review. Here are five that I think are important:

### 1. Safety:

Moving YLO into assisted living is a very personal and difficult decision but, with all the safety issues, you certainly don't want to second-guess yourself because you waited too long.

Things you might want to be concerned about: Oven, stove top, microwave, electrical hazards, heat and A.C. controls, dishwasher, clothes dryer, spoiled food, drinking enough/eating enough, medication issues, balance issues, sleeping too much/not enough, steps, lost keys, broken glass, accidents, emergencies... can YLO still use a telephone?

### 2. Behavior Problems:

Here is an email from Catherine:

> *As you know, Keith's situation has changed. He is a lot more agitated these days. He's taking his meds, too. One day I sat on the sofa all day because everything I tried to do – he would yell at me and tell me, "What are you doing???? This is NOT your house."*

You need to be prepared in case this happens. When the antipsychotic meds stop having an effect, then it can get very difficult (understatement) to live with someone. When the symptoms can't be controlled by medications anymore, then it's time to realize you are going to need help. This is the time when you look back and thank yourself for coming up with "a plan."

### 3. Incontinence:

"The 'accidents' are infrequent but we still can't take her out for fear of having one."

If someone can't go out of the house for fear of an accident, that is a game changer. Everyone is trapped. Changing underpants and pants every time is impossible. Judging when someone needs to use the bathroom is impossible. Freedom is diminished completely. It's a big, BIG deal. I had two clients that had incontinence issues and all our time was spent dealing with it. We weren't going to museums or out to lunch or visiting.

Now, because they live in assisted living, I ask the staff to take them to the restroom. A care manager will put on a new "pull-up" (adult diaper) and then we are out the door re-connecting with their "life."

### 4. Social Interaction:

A compelling reason to consider assisted living is the interaction that comes with the other residents, the staff and even the visitors. There is the potential for new friendships and new experiences.

### 5. You:

When I'm visiting one of my clients in assisted living I often see a worried and worn out son or daughter, husband or wife, on a "tour", looking for the right facility for their parent or spouse. I can almost sense the weight of their decision. Sometimes, I'd like to walk right up to them and say, *"You are getting this right. You are doing the right thing."*

You might think you are giving up if you place YLO in a "Home." You might think they deserve better, but right now, you need to look at the reality of the situation. Things must change. Your body and mind are breaking down. Alzheimer's is in total control.

Now is the time to let skilled professionals take care of YLO's needs because **you need help.** I tell this to the families I work with:

> *You are a very loving person. You will make the right decisions because of that. You have made some difficult decisions and now, here is the biggest one. When you are ready, make it and remember...*
>
> ***THE LUCKY ONES GET TO GO TO THESE PLACES!!!!!***

At the right time, assisted living can be a great fit. It can work out better than you expected. Great people, nice location, plenty of activities and access to nurses, doctors, dentists... and hairdressers! I'd live in a lot of these places and I have met some front-line staff, activities directors, and community directors who are the most wonderful people in the world.

And here is one of them.

**Interview with Darby (Continued from Pg. 135)**

Hello Darby! I have a few questions and I know you are the right person to ask.

Q.  (Henry) What are some important things that new residents and their families might need to know?

A.  *(Darby) With any kind of significant life change, there is often an overwhelming amount of things that people feel they need to know and understand. I like to make it as simple as I can for our new residents and their family members. The main thing that needs to be known is that their loved one is now in a safe place with a supportive environment that will, in most cases, improve the lives of the residents and produce positive and measurable outcomes. The residents and families need to know from the beginning that this is now the resident's new home, and the management and staff of the community are here to provide a safe and secure environment, offering the individual care and assistance that they need to remain at their optimal level of living, instead of simply surviving.*

Q.  What are the most asked questions from potential residences and their families?

A.  *Ah!! That is a loaded question in itself! There are so many questions that are asked in the initial conversations, so I will list some of the most frequently asked questions.*

*1. Obviously one of the first questions is about costs and contracts.*

*2. Another common question is, "At what point does the community initiate a discharge, or can my loved one remain in the community and be cared for through end of life?"*

*3. Does your community have a specialized memory care neighborhood?*

*4. What are the staffing patterns and ratio of staff to resident; for example, one care-giver to eight residents in memory care during the 6pm -2am shift?*

*5. What kind of personal care can you provide?*

*6. Can hospice services be brought into the community?*

*7. Are you regulated and licensed by the state?*

*8. What are the safety and security features in the community, and fire evacuation procedures?*

*9. What is your protocol if my loved one falls in the middle of the night?*

*10. Do you have nurses on staff?*

*11. Do doctors and other geriatric specialists come to the community?*

**Q.   What questions would you ask if you were moving your mom or dad into an assisted living facility?**

A.   *For me personally, my main question would be how does the community communicate with me, and how much? I would want to know who the point people are for different concerns and questions. I would want to know and be assured that the community has an adequate state survey that is current and hopefully free of violations, and I would ask for a copy. I would ask if I can have some contacts to call of other residents' family members to get an opinion from a third party who has moved in their loved one. I would ask, "How are you going to know if my mom or dad is not lying on the floor and what systems are in place in the event of emergencies?" I would ask about hydration and what system is in place. I would ask to see the kitchen and back hallways, so I can inspect the cleanliness from behind the scenes? I would also ask to have a private meeting with the executive director prior to making my decision.*

**Q.   Who is responsible for fingernails, toenails and personal grooming? Do you have someone who takes care of these or is that the responsibility of the family?**

A.   *In almost all cases, the personal care is done by the community. There will be a care plan in place for each resident. An on-site manicurist usually does fingernails, but there are certain conditions in which only a doctor can do cutting of fingernails, conditions such as diabetes, and residents on blood thinners. The toenails are done by a podiatrist, and most communities have a podiatrist who comes into the community about four times a year. Medicare covers the foot care cost.*

Q.   **What is protocol for dealing with an unruly resident with serious behavior problems or residents just not getting along? I know it's "involved" but this question is always on everyone's mind.**

A.   *Henry – You asked the question beautifully. When a resident starts to display serious behavior problems, intervention must happen right away. Often times, when someone develops a behavior change quickly, it is usually an acute situation the resident is experiencing such as a urinary tract infection, or a kidney infection. If those are not detected and treated right away, the resident will often become combative and display sudden increased confusion, and even at times hallucinations. So the community needs to have a system in place to immediately get the resident tested for an infection, and the medication needed to clear it up.*

*At other times the resident will start to have a change in condition due to the progression of the disease. Behavior issues can and do arise, and many times in-patient hospital stays are necessary to find out the best way to treat the resident and the behaviors. Often times, the resident may be in need of a medication change, or need to be put on a new medication. Most of the in-patient geriatric hospitals will keep the resident for a 10-to-14 day stay in order to adequately diagnose and prescribe treatment. Assisted living communities are not equipped to handle severe behavior issues on a daily basis, which is why it is important to have the resources and knowledge of who to contact when this occurs. Most assisted living communities will have a geriatric care specialist who follows the resident once back in the community after a hospital stay for behaviors, and they will come to the community for regular visits.*

**Q. What is the best feature about your facility for assisted living residents, and for memory care residents?**

A. *Again, a loaded question! We have so many wonderful features at my community. I would say one of our best offerings is our choice of non-drug therapy programs. Our company has done extensive research about alternative ways to handle the day-to-day "good, bad, and ugly" of the dementia resident. We use many different media including "Senses Therapy," which is designed to improve the quality of life using the five senses, Reminiscence therapies, cognitive stimulation therapies, animal and horticultural therapies, and many more. All of these provide those with Alzheimer's and other dementias the benefit of learning and mental activities to improve quality of life and functioning ability as prescribed from a non-drug therapy option.*

Thanks Darby! I know these answers will help a few families that are looking for the right place for their loved one. You are the best!

**"Your New Apartment!"**

Phrasing a change in living situations can make all the difference in the world. You may need to separate YLO's idea of assisted living, which is probably a combination of nursing home/haunted house, with what it really is – an apartment. Before the move you need to start talking about the new "apartment."

If you need to further explain this lovely apartment, use a few details. "Mom, it has a door you can close to the outside world. It will have your bed, your own bathroom, your dresser, your lamps and your pictures. You can control the temperature and you can open the shades. There are new friends to meet and plenty of activities that I know you will enjoy. This apartment is so nice!" Of course you might run into a brick wall of, *"Are you kidding me?"*

If the "new apartment" thing isn't working, use "With your new apartment I won't have to worry so much," or "I can't sleep any more knowing you are living alone," or if it's your spouse, it's safe to assume that conditions are untenable, so regardless of what they think, it has to happen.

My suggestion is to not let the comments "Are you kidding me" or "Please don't put me in a nursing home" discourage you from what needs to be done. Look forward and keep focused.

## Behavior Problems II

You know the brand new assisted living facility on the corner that looks like a giant Victorian mansion, lattice gazebo and all? Well, if YLO is "energetic" – to say the least! – this pretty, brand new, convenient facility might not be the right one. Just because it is an assisted living facility doesn't mean it's going to be the right place for YLO. You might have a hunch that the transition to assisted living might be very difficult for a number of reasons; one being that YLO will be highly motivated to NOT go there; second, there could be some behavior problems; third-they are mobile. Mobility with behavior problems can be a key issue.

The next ten pages are for families who know that although their loved one is not in a hurry to move they also know, in time, there is a good chance they might be accepting of their new home. If you think that YLO might have behavior issues talk to your doctor about the facilities in your area that might be able to handle a more "energetic" resident. If they don't know, ask them who does.

Just in case.

## How to Choose One

> The best way to determine the right assisted living facility for YLO is firsthand experience. This is how Mary Beth and I found the one for Mom – recommendations from friends. This next section offers you some direction should you not have any recommendations for a particular Home or there are just too many options to choose from.

Assisted living facilities really are different from one another. Different pricing, different care options. They are continuously changing because of the personalities of the different residents who move in and out. There is a lot to consider in deciding which one is best for YLO's needs.

Below are criteria that I think need to be met before you move YLO into an assisted living facility. I'm a bit harsh here, but I want what is best for you and YLO so I'm not going to hold any punches. **Most of these points are related to someone who needs assisted living/memory care and not skilled care.**

143

- Money: If there is not a lot of money then guess who's not going to the expensive Home? My mom had just enough money and an income where we could place her in a moderate Home with an outstanding reputation. Having or not having money will help you make a lot of these decisions.

- Budget (stick to it): With the help of a financial adviser/elder law attorney, set up a budget. What can you spend and how long will the money hold out? When you develop a budget, then it's time to visit the facilities that are within it. Some facilities are all-inclusive, however, some have extra fees (**a Care Plan**); ask if they have an annual price increase. Paying more in fees can mean more care for YLO – and that's a good thing, but make sure you understand the different pricing structures.

- Community Fee. A community fee (usually between 1K and 3K) is like a deposit, but not really – it is nonrefundable. So I guess it's like free money for the facility. How exciting! After hearing several vague definitions from facility managers about what this "fee" is for, the real problem is: What happens to that fee if YLO is asked to leave? This has been a tricky one for a few of the families I have worked with. More detail on this on page 214

- The staff: Ask the facility about their turnover rate. How many years have each of the front line staff/care managers (the people who actually feed, bathe, and work directly with the residents) been there? **This is important**. In poorly run homes you will see a huge turnover rate. No one wants to work there. If the staff doesn't want to be there, you don't want YLO there either. Don't let them off the hook by showing you two or three people who have worked there over ten years. Ask them about everyone who will be working with YLO.

- Reputation: Good or bad, they probably earned it.

- Aesthetics: No nice pictures, old carpet, no plants, no landscaping – if it looks like the owners are not concerned about the appearance, then you shouldn't be concerned about spending any money there. If they are not concerned about their residents seeing anything aesthetically pleasing or they think it's not important for the place to look nice, then I suggest you keep looking. Be aware that in some assisted living facilities, walking from the assisted living to the memory care is like night and day.

Here is a message I received from Harper, my client Marie's daughter.

Henry, I'm looking at the obvious and it took me forever to pick up on it. At both assisted living locations, the ambiance varied significantly for the memory care residents as opposed to the assisted living area. It gave me the impression the management may think "it doesn't matter" for the memory care residents, so no need to paint, have nice carpet, etc. And if this doesn't matter, what else doesn't matter? **I'd say she nailed it.**

- Vibe: A hippy word for sure but there is no better word that describes the overall feeling. When you walk in, how does it feel? When you are leaving, what comes to mind? Did you feel any uncomfortable pressure from the sales person? If you were the one with AD, could you see yourself living there?

- Space available: Ask how many beds or rooms are available. If the Home is half empty, that's probably a bad sign.

- Men: On average there is a 7:1 ratio of women to men in assisted living "communities" so it's no wonder that the decor and activities can feel a little "feminine." If you are looking for a facility for your father or brother ask about **specific activities geared towards men**. Also, look for one where a good percent of the population is male. Just ask for a current percentage. The presence of more men will likely influence the activity director towards "guy stuff." There might be more action; guys get into more trouble, they plan more, cut up more, and scheme more. We do; you ladies know it and you love it!

- Food: If you have a place in mind, set up an appointment at lunch time. Ask to see people having their lunch or maybe even ask if you can have lunch. Look around. Does the food look OK? Be careful using food or how it looks as a prerequisite in choosing a facility. You might have to cross out half your list. The chef might be having a bad day!

- Can I bring my dog?: At some of these places you can! Most of the places I go to have a community dog as well. I visit a client in a facility that not only has a dog, but they have birds, fish and a pig. No kidding. They have a micro-pot-belly piglet. Watching the dog Raven play with Piglet is something else!

- Activities: Entertainment, exercise, programs, fun things to do, the list goes on. The activities director in these homes is the person not sitting down. I remember one director brought in a belly dancer – the guys were on the edge of their seats. When you are scouting, check out the activity board and then see if these activities are actually taking place. The times are posted. If it says "Entertainment with Julie at 2:00", then at 2:00 check and see if Julie is entertaining. Julie might actually be *Love Boat* Julie and drinking a margarita with Isaac!

I was planning to place a client into assisted living and was given a budget and preferred location. The first one I walked into had a very nice chalk board loaded up with activities. I asked about the "Sunny Happy Walk" or whatever it was called. I thought "this is great!" The residents are actually getting out for a walk." Then I asked, "Where do you take them to walk?" She looked at me with a big smile and said, "It's a stroll through the front parking lot."

I am continuously blown away by what passes for an "activity" at some of these facilities and I think this makes a strong case for what I now believe – the activities director is the most important position in an assisted living facility. Here is an example why:

There are two facilities owned by the same company, sharing some of the same employees, in close proximity, same cost, same building age, same just about everything. The activities at one facility are hot dogs once a month in the courtyard, a drive every now and then, and maybe a birthday party – maybe.

At the other facility, it is Atlanta Braves ball games; trips to museums – even trips out of town; fishing for the guys; and lots of outings, drives, lunches and parties – real parties with live music and great participation from everyone. The staff takes suggestions from the residents' families about activities and makes them happen. It is astounding how much is going on there, and all because of one lady, the activities director. She is 100% engaged and her efforts are contagious. The atmosphere at the facility where she is employed is upbeat, happy and fun. It's always first on my recommendation list for anyone looking for memory care.

> *The other facility was just what you would expect from a Home... sleepy land. They were just getting by doing the bare minimum that the state of Georgia requires by law. **These places really are different.***

- Outings: Same as above. If there is an outing planned at 11:00 a.m. and the bus is still parked out front empty, ask why?

- Does it have a nursing wing for skilled care? I remember when my dad was looking for a Home for my grandmother; he was happy that the place he found had a nursing wing. She moved in to the retirement community, then moved over to the intermediate level, and eventually to the nursing wing. It was all on the same campus. The same was true with my mom. We didn't have to hire any extra care at the end like you would have to do at a place that didn't have a skilled care wing.

> *Do keep in mind that because of the different levels of care we have now, nursing homes are not your only option any more. There have been some changes over the years that now allow people to "age in place." Today many assisted living facilities have designated areas where people can get the extra help they need including skilled care and even hospice (end of life care).*

- Take a friend: I am not a shopper. When I go shopping, I don't buy anything. When my wife and I go shopping, I buy stuff. If finding a Home is a family effort, the more the merrier; everyone's input will be helpful. If it's just you, ask your best friend to come along with you when you are picking out a Home. They can remind you of the reality of the situation and guide you into committing to the right place. Your friend knows what's going on.

## The Move

You have carefully considered your options. You have walked into a facility that meets your criteria and even though you are anxious, you know it's the right thing to do. Depending on the facility, there are several steps you will need to take. For instance, YLO may need to be evaluated. This would entail the nurse on staff spending some time with YLO to observe, maybe over lunch or a walk around the facility. It's usually very informal. YLO might also have to go see his or her primary physician for a check up to make sure they are current on vaccinations. TB is the one they are most concerned about. If YLO is moving into memory care, you will need a dementia diagnosis from his or her physician. After you have signed about 600 pieces of paper (by now you will have probably memorized YLO's social security number), then it's time to move. Here is how I recommend doing this:

You can take YLO to see the new "apartment" building. Introduce YLO to the staff, a few new friends and have lunch. See if you can get a smile and if he or she feels comfortable. If so, in a few days have someone take YLO out for the day. While they are out, move. Hang their favorite pictures; bring their favorite pieces of furniture – everything that is their favorite, any detail that you can think of. Try and arrange everything the way they had it at home. This is not to fool them into thinking it's the same thing. It's just to make YLO's stay there as comfortable and as familiar as possible. Then take him or her over to the new apartment. This is the way we moved Mom. Not a pleasant memory, but I know it was the best thing for her.

The staff will have some great suggestions about moving and I also highly recommend you talk with someone at the Alzheimer's Association. I'm sure they will be able to give you the best advice knowing the details of your situation. There are companies that can help with the move and this transition if you think you might need the extra help. Also, some assisted living facilities have a "hotel room." YLO can spend the day/night there when you need a break or need to go out of town without YLO. It's also a good way to introduce (for some) a certain "community."

Here are a few reasons why, in my experience, the transition to assisted living has been so much better for most than everyone thought it would be.

- Although you might not have recognized it, your level of anxiety and stress directly affect and influence YLO. Being around family constantly or living at home alone can be stressful for YLO. He or she may put up a fight about moving, but once it's done, they might realize that this is what is best for them.

- Some people may be resistant to being told what to do in their home. (I wouldn't want someone in my house telling me what to do either). Since assisted living is neutral ground, YLO might become more responsive to "requests."

- The employees know how to get things done. These facilities are much better equipped in handling the various crises that can occur in some Alzheimer's patients.

- New friends: When we moved my client Marie into memory care she met "Marie from Switzerland" who also spoke French. They have been best friends from day one. My pals William and David had similar friendships develop almost immediately.

- There really is a big difference between an assisted living/memory care facility and a nursing home. I remember when we moved Mom into memory care, I met Carol, the music teacher. She played piano, taught music lessons and talked and visited with everyone. I thought "How great is this? A music teacher on staff." It took me three visits to realize she lived there! There are many residents who live in memory care because they just need a little help.

Take these points into consideration when you are having doubts about "the move."

There might be a period of "Why am I here?" and "Take me home please", and yes, that possibly could go on forever. However in most cases they know they are safe and there is always food on the table. You might even hear, "I like it here. Meet my new friend." After an initial few weeks, YLO might start to accept and make the best of the situation. It's not ideal but with AD, nothing is ideal. And of course, I have to keep saying it, this might be different from what you experience.

**You Picked One and YLO is Moved in. Now What?**

When you visit YLO the first few times, it's going be tough, especially leaving and saying goodbye. As time goes on, however, you will start to understand why this is the best situation for you both. Your life was so difficult before, but now, visiting with YLO might become enjoyable. I know this sounds like an ad, but it's true. Here are a few suggestions for what to do and what to expect.

- Getting out: Taking advantage of everything the facility has to offer is important, but taking YLO "out" is also important. Being able to leave depends on several factors, most importantly, can you get them back in... especially for memory care! Staff might recommend some settling-in time depending on how well YLO is accepting the new apartment, but after that, go. I have seen too many families just move their loved one into assisted living and that's it. No more trips. No more outings. Last week they went to church, this week they can't. Why? It's a little bit different for memory care, see page 157.

- Arrangements/Times: What time is your mom's favorite TV show on? Write them down (not all of them but the important ones) and tell the staff you would like them to make sure she is able to watch her favorite show. On a night where you have picked out a TV show for Mom to watch, show up unexpectedly to make sure your request is being taking care of. If she isn't watching her show, then you need to have a word with someone who is going to make that happen. These kinds of drop-ins keep everyone on their toes. You are not asking for the world – you just want your mom to see a few of her favorite programs every now and then. Small DETAILS are important! Example:

*My friend Ginnie loved Antiques Roadshow on PBS. For her it was the perfect show, all those heirlooms and antiques, with the explanation of what they are, how old, and how much they are worth – a great show for someone who has AD. No plot. The same could be said with sports: All action and no story. Travel and cooking shows are great too. Rick Steves is the best – a globetrotting gentle soul.*

- Show up at unexpected times: Most visits come around lunch or dinner, so occasionally show up at 8:30am or 7:00pm in the evening. I do it all the time. Again, it keeps everyone on their toes.

- Serving size: My mom ate like a bird. A big plate of food discouraged her from eating. It was too much. I quickly learned to serve her small portions so she wouldn't be overwhelmed. If you think this might be a problem for YLO, tell the staff to do the same. Understandably they have to follow certain guidelines but do not let them use that as an excuse for not using common sense.

- Companionship: I have seen several people move into assisted living/ memory care and after a year they have a new "special friend." My advice – be happy for them, but I'm not getting into all that romance stuff. Former Supreme Court Justice Sandra Day O'Connor has written extensively about this subject.

- Free Will: Your mom is independent and free to move about the Home as she chooses. There are plenty of things for her to trip over, just like at home, only with more space and more people to run into. When I moved Mom to memory care I thought, "Wait a minute, Mom could fall here. I thought this place was supposed to be safe?" Then I realized the only other option would be for her to stay in bed possibly heavily medicated.

  *People actually fall in assisted living more than they do at home, but you can't always blame the staff for someone falling. It's just not possible to watch forty people interacting, walking up and down the hall and in their rooms. These places are mini worlds and you don't want your dad strapped to a bed, so you have to let go a bit. Be prepared to see a few Band-Aids.*

- Others like yourself: If I showed up between 2:00 and 4:00 any day of the week at the Lowman Home where Mom lived, I knew I would see Tom. He was there every day visiting his wife Gail. Through his caring nature and deep devotion to her, he taught me so much about life and helped me cope with what I was going through with Mom. Tom was always sweet to Mom and always engaged her, "Hello Sandra, how are you today?" or "You look so pretty in that blouse…" Any small effort he made to keep an eye on her was very important to me. I try and do the same. The more eyes on YLO, the more "Hellos" they receive, the better you will sleep. There are plenty of "yous" in each facility and it's to your advantage to develop a good support system between you all.

This is why:

Here is an email I sent to Tiffany; she is a manager at a memory care facility.

*Hey Tiffany,*

*Henry here, Karen's friend. I like the new train set idea. Looking forward to watching it.*

*Last week I noticed Charles was having a lot of trouble eating his lunch. Most of it ended up on the floor. No one assisted him. Today I noticed the same thing. He was trying to cut his meat with a spoon. I waited until lunch was almost over and still – no help offered from the staff. I borrowed a knife, found another fork and helped him eat. I could tell he really appreciated it. He seemed relieved that someone cared. I asked the care-manager who was standing 6 feet away why no one offered to help him out and she had no answer. Matter of fact, she seemed to resent the question.*

*If I see this happen again I am going to notify his family and maybe a few other people.*

*Just wanted to let you know.*

*Thanks Tiffany,   Henry*

If you have a grievance or see something that just doesn't seem right, there is protocol: The facility might have a form you can fill out. Also, as you develop relationships with some of the staff (naturally you might gravitate toward a few) you can always just mention to them what your concerns are. A phone call to one of the facility's managers might do the trick as well.

"Please help Charles cut up his food" was such a simple, solvable problem. I was angry and I saw a pattern developing. It should have been obvious to everyone in the room that he was having trouble. Maybe this wasn't an emergency, and to some this might seem insignificant but, for Charles it wasn't.

*I had a hard time making contact, but I felt this problem demanded immediate attention. I took a different route – it worked. Problem solved.*

---

Start a network with the other residents, families and friends so you can share information and observations. Swap email addresses and phone numbers. Work together in making sure the level of care YLO's are receiving is appropriate. The more people looking out for YLO the better off he/she will be. **As consumers we have the power to make a difference.**

---

- Have a plan B: It's just not working out at a particular home. The staff is slow at responding to requests and questions you have. Maybe a larger corporation has just bought the Home and they have decided to let half the staff go, unfortunately the half you like. There is no trust, and you don't feel comfortable having YLO live there. Well, pack their bags and move. For the money you are paying, you should expect a great relationship with the staff and a rapid response to your concerns. No exceptions. If they don't have the time for you and your concerns, this is a clear indication that it's time to go.

**And on the flip side – Having a plan B is also important if YLO has been asked to move.** That can happen. Too many brush ups. Too confrontational. Too many physical altercations with other residents and the staff. If this happens, as Darby said, there is protocol.

### Developing a Fall Plan

For a minute let's pretend you have AD and live in an assisted living facility. Alicia (CNA) walks in and sees you on the floor of your room. 911 is called. The paramedics show up, you are put on a stretcher, lifted into an ambulance, and driven to the hospital. You are probably in some pain and thinking "Where are we going?" You arrive at the hospital and are asked a series of questions, a few prods and pricks of a needle. Lots of people in green uniforms with name tags. "Am I in a hospital? This is where sick people go."

There is no doubt that hospitals, doctors and nurses do a tremendous job. Hospitals give life. But hospitals zap life too. The event that happened (something traumatic), a fall, maybe surgery. Mentally things might start to become unhinged. If you are in bed for three days, leg muscles go unused; the level of stress is high; the lack of routine, unfamiliar surroundings, add to it all. This event could possibly add to YLO's general cognitive decline.

Some assisted living facilities don't have enough staff for someone to ride along in the ambulance and answer all the questions at the hospital so you need to make arrangements in case you can't be there. Here are a few other suggestions:

- Make sure the hospital staff knows to give certain medications at certain times. There is a different nurse every eight or twelve hours and different doctors for different procedures. With so many rotating people, something is bound to get missed and when some of my people skip their anti-psychotic meds, trouble is just around the corner. You don't need to be worrying whether your dad was administered his meds (he is in a hospital!) You need to make the case that is it very important "for this drug to be administered at this time."

- TV, books and magazines are about the only friends you have, so use them to the fullest. Tell the staff, "Dad likes to watch ESPN." A loved TV show is comforting. Lower YLO's anxiety by any means you have.

- Hospitals can discharge anyone when they think their responsibility has been met. Here is how it works: Your mom fell, has four broken ribs, and a partially collapsed lung, but now, three days later, "She is fine. Come and get her."

   ...What?

Sometimes you have to fight for care. No one at the hospital has any idea of what YLO was like before they arrived. You do. Tell them what you expect to happen before YLO is discharged. Most people are assigned a case worker. That is your "go to" person. Make sure you are in contact with them for any questions. They are the ones who talk with the doctors and nurses and will help you make a few decisions. They can even help you line up a physical therapy/rehab facility and transportation.

## Skilled Care: Physical Therapy Facility/Rehabilitation Center

Let's keep pretending...

During your hospital stay the doctor suggested going to a rehab center for physical therapy (PT) to help you get your strength back before going home or back to "The Home." (Most assisted living facilities have some sort of PT but it's not as intensive as an actual PT facility).

If your hospital stay is for three days or more, Medicare usually pays 100% for the first twenty days and an additional eighty co-pay days. (Elder Law territory!) That's good for you. But naturally with this system, and of course this is my opinion, the high prices rehab facilities charge for care (what **WE ALL** end up paying for) are way out of sync with the services they provide.

I have been to six rehab facilities and they all look the same to me. Not many pictures on the walls. The rooms are small. No frills. It makes a stay at the hospital look like Disney World. The hard work, personalities and capabilities of the staff are what make any of these places successful and they do work hard trying to get people moving again. I look at these places as a sort of boot camp; you go there to go to work, a short stay place, hopefully. The mornings are like a beehive of activity. Physical therapy (PT) is usually exercises. I used to think occupational therapy (OT) was a big word for blocks and puzzles, but I was way off. It can also include how to get dressed, help with grooming, and setting up a system for a resident with signs reminding them of what not to do or what to do, (for example, "Throw paper towels in this trash can" with an arrow pointing down to the trash can), etc. In some facilities there isn't much going on over the weekends, but come Monday the action begins. Three hours of PT, OT, then lunch and maybe another round. I don't think there is much of a difference between these places. I'm sure the various facility employees would have a heart attack at that statement.

The food: The places I have been to should be embarrassed by what they serve. Rehab means trying to get better, right?

Everyone is going to have a different experience and I'm trying not to be discouraging, but as you can probably tell, these places are without a doubt my least favorite of all the skilled care facilities. I have been disappointed too often to not say anything. It's sort of a catch 22. Without these facilities; it's the hospital or home, so rehab centers are vital and very necessary. I just think for the price *we all pay* – they should be a lot better.

Recently, I walked into one and my client hadn't been served his dinner. It was 8:00 p.m. He was there because of an intestinal infection that just would not go away. We had no clue if they were actually feeding him or giving him his medicine. Somehow he had gotten lost in the shuffle. $9,000.00/month is a lot to pay to get lost in the shuffle. We actually had to hire a sitter so the family would know he was getting his medicine. Isn't that bizarre? A guy moves into skilled care/rehab facility and the family has to hire someone to make sure he is being taking care of? You might want to take a look at a few before deciding where to go.

**Getting the Most Out of a Rehab Center**

To maximize the benefit, be proactive at getting the most out of rehab for YLO.

- Make sure YLO participates and is involved in all the activities offered at the facility. Sometimes they are a little slack in getting everyone involved so you need to bend someone's ear and make sure your mom is involved. Sign her up for everything you think she might enjoy.

- Get that hair washed! I don't mean to harp on the hair and nails but I have noticed that you really have to get on the staff at some of these places to get it done. Toenails that are too long – don't want to discourage walking at ALL in a rehab center! Sorry to go on and on about these, but I just see it everywhere I go. It's such an obvious sign of neglect.

- Since it is a place where people go to work to get better, you can't be disruptive. I received this message from the son of one of my clients.

  *The OT nurse told me on Friday that Dad had grown increasingly belligerent during the week, refusing to try anything she was trying to teach him. They planned to discharge him this Thursday. I am very hopeful that his calmer demeanor now will encourage them to keep him longer. OT will let us know tomorrow.*

Anything you can do to help YLO feel as relaxed as possible can be very important to their progress.

Small improvements everyday will add up and these places can work miracles. I have seen people wheeled in and then walk out. My suggestion; as an advocate for YLO, stay on your toes, keep your eyes open, and bring in some real food every now and then.

## Memory Care

I am very thankful for memory care. I can't imagine our world without it. It is a safe environment and understandably it's quieter than assisted living with less activities and outings. There are many reasons someone with advanced dementia can't stay at home but just like any transition it can vary from person to person. Usually, after a while, everything clicks and the wheels keep turning.

But... things can go haywire.

When we moved my client Steve into memory care, it was a pretty rough transition. His family was reluctant to let the nurse on staff administer any medications that might make him sleepy. I remember both his daughter and son saying, "We don't want him drugged-up."

Now if Steve was confined to a wheelchair the accommodation might have been possible, but Steve was still highly mobile (he was everywhere!) and that can make things difficult.

### Mobility + Aggressive Behavior + Everywhere = TROUBLE

Well shortly after the move, Steve was asked to leave. He was too difficult to care for.

The family didn't want him zonked out. The staff found it impossible to care for him. I understand both sides. The problem might have been solved by finding some middle ground. In my opinion, medication is and should be used to ground someone. If it works and lowers the level of anxiety, fear and unhappiness, maybe their life will be more peaceful. That's what I would want.

I'm sure there are many instances where the staff has over-prescribed meds. No denying that. If everyone is "easy breezy", it's less work. However, in my experience, with a doctor and nurse supervision, caring staff members and participation from the family, the right meds can offer life again... real life.

Most families understand that for the safety of every one medications are necessary but – even with all the various medicines it can still be a huge challenge for some families finding a memory care facility for their loved one who has behavior problems. I'm not sure why there are no facilities designed like a long term stay psychiatric hospital "for a reasonable price", (or at the very least how about a facility someone can go that can help with the transition?) It's a black hole in our healthcare system and one of the main reasons for so much of the anxiety. I am not sure why we don't have a better answer.

**Outings in Memory Care**

I use routine and repetition to get my clients out and about. Assisted living facilities also use them (sometimes a bit too much!) But I understand... These are important tools used get things done. When you move YLO into memory care the staff might discourage you from outings. This is what I recommend: **Use Your Own Judgment.** If YLO has acclimated well, has a few friends and you are able to get them back into the facility without too much coaxing, then keep taking them out. But if YLO is not adjusting well and after the outing it's hard to get them to settle or, after you drop them off, the staff has a very difficult time calming YLO down – then outings are not a good idea. This understanding is best for YLO.

**One Last Point About Choosing an Assisted Living Facility**

I think the most important observation you can make when you are scouting an assisted living facility, whether it's memory care or skilled care (especially a nursing home), is to try and take a look at everyone living there. Some of these people might not ever get a visit from family or friends; they might have moved from a different state or might not have an advocate or anyone to observe what kinds of care they are receiving. If they look like they are not being taken care of, then you might expect similar care for YLO.

Keep in mind some of the pretty facilities might be rotten on the inside and some of the older, not so pretty ones might be wonderful. Pay attention to all the details: Unwashed hair, bad smells, people wandering around half dressed – all obvious signs that someone is not being taken care of.

Just think about how important it is to someone who has lived their whole life where they care about their appearance and now, they have no control over what they wear, how they look, the condition of their fingernails, whether they bathe. What if no one will help you cut up your food?

**Some "small" missed detail is not small at all if it's –**

# you.

# Part 3.

# A Few Minor Adjustments

## BINGO and Led Zeppelin

Last year I received a call from a lady who was looking for help for her husband who had AD. I was asking about his interests and she said right up front her husband's favorite band was Led Zeppelin.

"Did you say Led Zeppelin?"

If we do the math some of these men and women who have early onset Alzheimer's are in their 50s and early 60s. That would put some of them in their teen-age years in the mid to late 1960s. In 1968 the Top 40 was The Doors, The Stones, Hendrix, and James Brown (The Godfather). Elvis had his comeback in '68.

I was visiting my pal Gene (my very first client) at his assisted living home and they had a sing along planned. Two ancient hippies showed up with acoustic guitars and started up with some lame rendition of "Don't Worry, Be Happy".[2] Gene started laughing and then ran for the exit. He couldn't say it, but I knew what was going on in his mind: He could not believe his life had come to this.

If your generation's music was The Clash or Earth, Wind and Fire, you might not be into acoustic guitars and sing-a-longs. Some of these guys were cops, or in the Marine Corps and you are telling me some music group called The Joy Express is going get everyone to sing and clap? Not going to happen. I hope some changes are made before I get there because I'm pretty sure I won't want to be singing "Don't Worry, Be Happy".

... Real sure.

## Changes

I'm not advocating playing Zeppelin in nursing homes, but I am suggesting that with a few minor adjustments, these Homes could be a little more "welcoming" to the next generations. Here are a few I recommend:

- Nurse outfits? Who wants to live in a hospital?

- I mentioned earlier in the section "Adult Day Care" about "Groupings." From observations in assisted living facilities most of the time everyone is together all day long. If they do split into groups it's generally men in one group and women in the other. That's about it. That's the grouping. Again, the groupings should be considered on their cognitive abilities, similar interests and similar personalities.

How about this:

1. Travel club: Those who are interested in getting together and talking about traveling. Watch travel videos, look at pictures and swap stories. (Dogs, traveling, movies, plans, walking. Guilty!)

2. Movie club: Instead of watching *Abbott and Costello Meet the Mummy* (again), how about a Steve McQueen movie?

3. Baking club: For those who would like to bake a cake or cookies.

4. Walking club: Get out for a walk every day in the neighborhood or take the community bus to a park. Key words – **EVERY DAY.** Sorry, but a stroll over some black asphalt in the front parking lot is lame.

5. Art club: Art appreciation through books, video and trips to museums and galleries.

6. Sports club: Sports on TV, vintage videos, trips to ball games.

Etc...

I might catch some heat from a few assisted living facilities by saying these because they do offer different activities, but do they encourage everyone to attend? Nope. Just because they offer it doesn't mean your mom will be there. I think a "club" environment with a specific time – where you would sign YLO up – would help everyone know who is supposed to attend.

Also, even if YLO can't participate, they still might enjoy being there.

- More Marvin Gaye AND Tammy Terrell. More Otis Redding, Motown, Stax, Beach Music, British Invasion. Jazz: Monk, Parker, Coltrane and Davis, and, of course, Herb Alpert. How about some pre-1979 Aerosmith, Sly and Robbie (to cool things out) or Curtis Mayfield – well, maybe not those just yet, but how about along with *Lawrence Welk*, they could add *Dick Clark, American Bandstand?* It might be helpful for all of us to remember that everyone who is 60-plus used to be 17.

- A meaningful existence with purpose (in a memory care facility). There are plenty of people who live in these Homes who are ready to go to work just like they have their whole lives. Now they do nothing for themselves. Some can't, I understand, but some of them can and they might want to. Put them to work; folding their laundry, setting the table, doing the dishes, sweeping their room, watering plants, dusting, etc. Just a few tasks that would be beneficial for them and the "community." Would some of the residents resent washing the dishes? You bet. But I think with a more robust emphasis on getting the residents who would like to do a few more things for themselves, to participate in these tasks, would in turn enhance their lives. I also understand that it would be time consuming for the staff, but would be worth it – well, maybe not worth it for the shareholders, but certainly worth it to the people who live there.

- "The Chalk Board Shuffle." Instead of a long list of "activities" that might or might not happen throughout the day, have a shorter list of a few quality ones that will.

- More activities outside when the weather is nice. Sunshine = Vitamin D. Most assisted living/memory care facilities have a nice courtyard – use it.

- "A Professional Visitor." The memory care facility could hire someone to come and visit with every resident. That would be their job – just to visit. *"You are important to me right here, right now."* They would spend ten to fifteen minutes a day with everyone in the building. They could have a folder for each resident with favorite pictures and photos, topics of conversation and interests, and talk about their "history." They would visit and send an email to the primary care-giver relaying what they said, or did that was interesting. Also, they could make sure the residents' needs are being taken care in a more personalized manner.

... Just suggestions for the "suggestion box".

## Food (Again)

Now, I'm not a *foodie* at all but I just can't write a section about assisted living and not make a few "comments" about the food.

There is more of a connection with the staff and residences in an assisted living/memory care facility than say at a "rehab facility" or hospital, so they tend to care a little more about what they serve. The higher end assisted living facilities will of course have better food and more options. You get what you pay for. Some operate just like a restaurant, made to order. In most of the assisted living facilities I go to (the moderately priced ones), it's hit or miss. Some of the food looks and tastes pretty good and some of it looks like what they served us at Forest Lake Elementary.

I see lots of casseroles and meat loaf and I guess that's all fine, but is it really that hard to take a handful of fresh spinach, put it in a pan, sauté with a little olive oil and squeeze of lemon? Or bake a potato? How about sliced tomatoes in the summer? Atlanta is surrounded by farms (none of which grow good peaches) but I just don't see much "fresh" anything. Some of these facilities sure could use a little help from my dietician pal, Corinne.

Maybe in a few years this will all change when the Baby-Boomer-Whole-Foodies start showing up in big numbers with their discerning tastes, but for now, I can't blame the residents for occasionally being a little disappointed in their dining experience.

## Back to School

One rainy afternoon I was visiting a client in a memory care facility and was looking for something to do. I happened to glance over at a book shelf in the activities room and saw a group of DVDs called "Museum Masterpieces" (a set of DVDs based on a college course on the *Louvre*)[3].

"Why not?"

I invited a few of her pals to watch but wasn't quite sure what I was getting everyone into. Well, by the end of the first hour not only did we have our original four watching, there were five others who joined us. Everyone was sitting quietly and watching intently. I couldn't believe it.

Most of these people were struggling with normal day-to-day tasks, but something about the seriousness and the scholastic approach seemed important enough to watch. This wasn't an hour-long documentary about the art collection in the *Louvre*. This was a class taught by a professor that included intense detail and technical analysis on a few paintings at the *Louvre*. It was a real lecture and, if this had been high school, everybody would have been asleep. The DVDs were probably donated by some "optimistic" person, but they had never been opened. The staff asked me if they were mine.

These nine people who lived in a memory care facility were all connected to something vital – a challenging scholastic exercise. We were all in school, learning.

I think this is relevant because even though someone's thought process might be interrupted by AD, we still need to respect the human mind. We all strive to maintain our connection to learning and self-improvement so serious mental stimulation is important, whatever the subject matter, (mathematics, history, music, science and nature, fine arts). This exposure, even in the later stages of AD, is not only respectful of their minds, but can greatly enhance their lives. I think a little more PBS and a little less junk TV would, along with the other "adjustments," help break some of the stigmas associated with assisted living.

# Part 4.

# Why I Really Like Assisted Living

Most of the people who work in assisted living facilities are really wonderful and very caring. I can be a little critical of Homes but I don't have a clue how to run one. It's usually 40 to 60 people living together with limited supervision. Packs are "forged." Lunch pals bond. Socially, it's high school all over again. I loved high school so maybe that's why I like assisted living. That might be an important factor to consider while reading this.

There is good and bad with any assisted living facility, but it has been my experience that a lot of these places are truly exceptional. You just have to find the right one. You have to participate, and you have to be an advocate for YLO. Even though you placed YLO in their care, your job is not over. You have to follow through and constantly make sure the job the facility has agreed to do (taking care of YLO) is being done. Along the way, and this is just my opinion, I believe it is everyone's responsibility to make sure **all** of the residents are being taken care of. First and foremost, I am an advocate for my clients, but I am also an advocate for everyone who lives there. We are all in this together.

Are there problems? Sure, all of them have their problems, but it's a big task and I think most of these places have way more pluses than minuses. Most days, there are planned activities and places to go. Girls Scouts drop by with hugs and cookies; parties, events, happenings and movies. There are religious services, and yes, even a few "sing-a-longs." It can be fun, exciting, and rewarding in many ways, and most of the staff works hard to make the lives of their residents better.

And this is why I love them...

### Mom's Friend Pat

After Mom was diagnosed, she did pretty well on her own. At times, it seemed as though the advance of the disease had temporarily halted. She had long plateaus where there were no big changes and no noticeable differences. But gradually things did start to change. She grew more confused and certainly needed more help. We all agreed it was time to place her in a Home. I remember the first time I took her to the Lowman Home for a visit:

163

We were having lunch with the residents and she pointed her finger around the room and said, "Is this me?"

When I moved Mom into the Lowman, she wasn't that thrilled to be there. It took a while before she got used to the idea of living in a dorm. She did have a nice room to herself and there was a nurses' station just down the hall and plenty of potential new friends, but she was a loner. I know she would have rather been at home, but that just wasn't possible any more. She was depressed that it had come to this.

*... And then came Pat.*


Oh my, did Pat look like a handful. Lots of adjectives I could use but I'll just say she was colorful inside and out. When I first met Mom's new friend, I thought, "What have I gotten Mom into?" Mom was a lady in every sense of the word. She was very sophisticated without being a snob. She was accepting of everyone just so long as they were polite and had a few manners. Pat, well, Pat had everything in spades.

After the initial shock I realized that Pat was actually sent by God. No kidding. Pat was there to meet and help Mom, and Mom was there to be her best friend. I have known Pat for nearly ten years. I still keep in touch and go see her every now and then. She helps everyone wherever she is. Everyone. The world needs more Pats.

Mom and Pat became best friends overnight. They were never separated. The staff called them the Bobbsey Twins. She had Mom over to her apartment (room) all day, every day, watching movies, visiting and talking. Mom had Pat on a walking regimen. They went everywhere together. Pat didn't have dementia. She had had a nervous breakdown while she was taking care of her mom who did have Alzheimer's. Pat was shipped from Florida to South Carolina on a bus in an almost comatose state. She had gotten better due to sheer perseverance and was now the life of the party.

We (Mary Beth, Poochie, Mom's friends, and myself) all started talking about Pat. It was so wonderful to have her as Mom's new best friend. I didn't worry so much! Those two had the strongest bond possible. Having Pat as her best friend gave Mom an extra year in her nice apartment; otherwise she would have had to transfer to the memory care unit. Pat would come and get Mom for every meal if they weren't already together. (If you can't get to dinner then that is a sign you need to be transferred to memory care). Pat would get Mom for all the activities and all the trips –

Pat was involved with everything possible that the Lowman had to offer and right next to her was my mom.

Wonderful. Wonderful! How wonderful!!!!!!!

Pat was Mom's last best friend who she met on her own. I love you, Pat. You are a gift to the world.

Especially mine.

# Overwhelmed

# 11.

When Mom was diagnosed with Alzheimer's, I didn't know anything about care-giving. Nothing. I had one plant on top of my refrigerator that I had pulled out of a trash can. That was the extent of my "care-giving." I didn't have a clue about what to do, where to go, or how to ask for help.

In the years that followed, I came to know that this dreadful disease was unlike any that I could have ever imagined. AD essentially attacks one's mind and inside the realm of that mind is who we are. As a care-giver, I constantly felt helpless. I could not help her in ways that I thought I should have been able to.

**Watching my mom struggle through this disease for so long
is where Alzheimer's really took its toll.**

Now, when I look back, I do think my Mom and I had it somewhat easy compared to some of the families I work with. Mom had a little emergency money tucked away, which allowed us the luxury of assisted living. She was so sweet and never uncooperative. We had great support from our family and friends. Personally, I had a lot of support from my wife Darcy (I'm not quite sure I would have made it through without her), as well as the incredible amount of help I received from my dad, Henry Sr. and stepmother Martha. They all understood what Mom and I were going through and supported me tremendously in every way. But, I still worried all the time. I had serious doubts about my ability as a care-giver and that continued for all eight years. At times I think I did all right but somehow it was still inadequate. Not a day goes by that I don't think I could have done a better job as a care-giver, but the more I do this and the more care-givers I meet, the more I realize that everyone feels this way. Dementia is just bigger than you are. It is a huge challenge.

When people ask me what I do for a living, I say "I work with people who have Alzheimer's." As we talk, I tell them what I do, how it works, why it works and, occasionally, if I have sounded like I know a thing or two, they may ask me, "Any advice?" And then I say, "The most important thing I can tell a care-giver is... Your loved one does not want you to worry so much."

Some people understand what I am saying. Some people look at me like (as if to say), "That's the big idea?"

Yes. That's the big idea. If you take one thing away from this book, I hope it's this one. If my mom knew how much I worried, she would have had a fit. Our loved ones with Alzheimer's want the best for us. The last thing in the world they want is for us to worry ourselves sick.

I remember one Christmas time when Mom was in assisted living, I picked her up and we were going to write Christmas cards together. I was racing around town with her in the car, trying to find cards, buying stamps, looking for lunch, trying to visit a few of Mom's friends, tracking down addresses. I needed to drive back to Atlanta that night and we had so much to do. I was stressed, tired, completely worn out. The constant worrying was really getting to me.

I was either working or driving to see Mom. Well, that day we were having no fun. If I had been able to think more clearly, we could have had a nice time, but I had run myself ragged. I had been exhausted for a few years and had worried myself into a depression. Just ask my friends. I very rarely saw any of them. I didn't make the time.

Four or five years after Mom was diagnosed, I started to get really bad headaches. Not ordinary headaches but the kind of headaches that made me sick. I saw a doctor and he said I was having migraines compounded by an old neck injury. I was under so much stress that toward the end of Mom's life, my body just started to fall apart. It has been seven years now since she died and I am just now starting to mend. I wish I had made it a priority to take care of myself and to keep what was happening in perspective. She would have wanted that.

At some point as a care-giver you might feel; stress, anxiety, worry, depression, irritability, sadness, exhaustion, anger, fatigue, fear and loneliness. Of course you will. **You have the toughest job on the planet.**

If you can, take a trip – without YLO. Ask for help from family and friends who can relieve you from constant care-giving, so you can get away. I know you might feel guilty, but do it. It will refresh you and make you a better care-giver. You need to try to take quality breaks from time to time because Alzheimer's is constant; it's always there, so try to find those hours for your own sanity and health.

In working with my clients, I've seen many people struggle to balance life and caregiving. Looking at some specific challenges might help you sort through your own situation and see it more clearly.

Patricia's husband has moderate-to-advanced stage AD. She works forty five to fifty hours a week. In the morning she wakes up and gets ready for work, then gets Mike ready. She makes breakfast while trying to get everything in order, arranging a care-giver for Mike while she is gone. Mike is becoming more delusional and his AD is progressing. Last week Patricia had a call from a neighbor because Mike was just wandering around the neighborhood. She needs to be focused at work, but worries constantly. After work, she drives home, cooks, and provides the entertainment for Mike, exhausted. She still expends the energy to communicate with him, even though he can't really complete a sentence. She then tries to get him to sleep, although he is restless. She wakes up and does it all over again, every single day. The man she lives with now is so different from the man she married. She hasn't received an anniversary gift or a birthday card from Mike in years. *She is devastated knowing he is never going to get better.*

And there's Sam. Sam's wife, Susan, has dementia. He is not getting much help from the kids or from Susan's sister. He looked into a day care, but the one he wanted to get her into was full. They both had to take early retirement and their savings is evaporating. He hasn't been able to play golf or go fishing in months because he can't find anyone to stay with Susan. Their friends don't stop by anymore because her behavior is very unpredictable. Sometimes she's a sweetheart, but other times she is a tiger.

Beverly has early stage Alzheimer's, and her children all live far from home. When her husband, Robert, asks them for help, they say, "Well, Dad, Mom sounds fine when she is on the phone with me." The kids see no need to worry so much. When they do come home, some of Beverly's symptoms seem to temporarily subside, which is something that frequently happens when early stage AD sufferers have visitors. But when the kids leave, Beverly's symptoms return and Robert feels frustrated and alone.

### Disappearing Friends

Alzheimer's is the "silent disease." No one wants to talk about it and everyone is scared of it. The word "Alzheimer's" is terrifying. That is why everyone avoids the issue and the main reason why we don't take our loved ones to see a neurologist. We don't want to hear the word ALZHEIMER's. (The golden years that were supposed to be filled with traveling, visiting and relaxing are not going to happen as you planned). On top of this is an effect that AD has on certain family members and lifelong friends. I see it all the time. Best friends turn into fair-weather friends and some family members just disappear; men are especially guilty. It's sad to see lifetime friends just stop coming for visits when their best pal has AD. I even know a few sons out there who avoid going to see their fathers, and daughters who avoid their mothers. A few years ago, a son of one of my clients told me "It just makes me too sad to visit Dad." I very diplomatically reminded him that this wasn't about "him" and that his dad really wanted to see his son.

I remember a few of my mom's pals completely disappeared after she was diagnosed. I thought "Where is so-and-so? They know Mom is sick. Are they going to come and see her?" Nope. They never did. They didn't even pick up the phone.

I think it's important for everyone to know what's happening so they can plan to come and visit periodically. Then the changes will be more gradual and less shocking. Using some discretion, maybe tell a few friends that YLO's memory is not what it used to be and visiting would be so beneficial. Maybe even make a few suggestions about how they could spend some time together, which might make a difference. It might not but I think making an effort and doing what you can to help maintain YLO's lifelong friendships, even as Alzheimer's progresses, will keep an encouraging support system intact not only for YLO, but also for you as a care-giver.

There are many reasons why someone might not be participating. For younger people or someone who has never lost anyone close or experienced overwhelming grief and sadness, it might take longer for them to realize the restrictions of time. Or, maybe someone doesn't know quite what to do – they might need some help finding their value. Some family members might be good with finances and numbers, some might be better at care-giving or making difficult decisions. Some might be great at lifting spirits with their sense of humor – very important. Alzheimer's has a quiet sadness that is impossible to describe so **humor, good cheer and laughing are more important than just about anything.** Everyone might have something valuable to offer, friends included, so I wouldn't count someone out because they seem distracted or unconcerned. It's worth a try.

## Getting Help

Towards the end of Mom's life, the last, best thing I did for her, and for ME, was to hire Lisa. Lisa was a CNA care-giver who would come over three or four times a week for about two hours at a time. She lived across the street from the Lowman Home so she could split up her visits as she chose. She was an incredibly loving person – a natural. I had gotten to a point where I needed someone else to help look after Mom; someone to be her friend, just like what people need when they hire me now. I felt so much better knowing Lisa was there to help.

At this late stage of AD, I was concerned with Mom getting enough to eat. She really started to lose weight. She couldn't use a fork anymore and grabbing food with her hands had become difficult. She needed a little help getting in and out of chairs. Mom needed help with just about everything.

Lisa helped her finish her food, did her nails, held her hand for hours and helped her interact with the other residents. Lisa was inspired. She was wonderful with Mom. Lisa is a genuinely gifted care-giver. She talked to Mom, put makeup on her and brushed her hair. Lisa would call me after almost every visit. I can't even begin to tell you how much that meant. At this point, I was so worried about Mom I felt awful all day. But when I got the calls from Lisa, I felt a lot better. She helped me through so much and just knowing she was there made me feel less overwhelmed.

Lisa, the love you showed Mom will always be appreciated. I can't ever thank you enough.

## A Very Special Dinner

Even in the later stages of AD, I would take Mom out for a good steak. I'd ask for a booth so she could sit next to me. Mom was almost a vegetarian but, man, did she love a steak every now and then. I would order one and we would split the salad and potato. I'd help her with her fork, cut her meat. The people sitting around us would look over every now and then. It's not normal to take someone who can't use a knife to a steak restaurant.

Were we disturbing these people trying to enjoy their meals? Were they uncomfortable seeing the reality of Mom's disease up close? Was it wrong for me to be bringing Mom into this restaurant in her condition? I wasn't sure if what I was doing was the right thing.

One evening something happened that remains one of my happiest moments during the whole time my mother was sick. I was having dinner with Mom at this steakhouse, and a lady walked behind our table. Then she walked around to see me, she looked at Mom. She stopped and looked right at me with a warm smile and gave me the thumbs up, with both hands, as if to say, "You go, boy! You are doing the right thing!"

Throughout the whole time, I wish I could have felt better about the job I was doing. A few people told me I was getting it right but I wasn't listening. This lady helped me realize that yes, my "get out and go" approach was exactly what Mom wanted, to keep getting out to enjoy a good meal, to see a friend, to see movies – to see the world, right up until the end. Instinctively, I knew it was the right thing but it just wasn't normal. It was such a sad time for Mom and me, and for this one stranger to validate what I was doing was one of the most comforting things I have ever experienced. Yes, I was making the right decisions.

You're damn right I was doing the right thing.

You are probably anxious and worried like I was, but I just bet you are an outstanding care-giver. Do you know how I know that? Because you are a very loving person. The decisions you are making are based on your love for that person. It's the restrictions that are to blame, not your decisions. I know you are exhausted and you are giving it all you have but as long as you are honoring YLO with every decision, you are doing the right thing even though it might not feel that way. When you are the primary care-giver, it feels like the weight of the world is on your shoulders but you are not alone thinking that way – I had no idea what I was doing. We are all amateurs at this. You have probably never been a care-giver before so it's OK to not know what you are doing. It's OK to feel inadequate and helpless. What's not OK is for you not to ask for the help and support you need to get through this difficult challenge.

**You always need to remember – our loved ones appreciate everything we have to give, even if they are not able to express that.**

AD had brought me to easily the lowest point in my life, but that lady's gesture is such a happy memory. I know she probably never realized how much it meant, but at that time… it meant the world.

## My Friend

The Reverend Howard Maltby is one of my best pals and has been a friend of the family for over ten years. He conducted Mom's funeral service and, let me tell you, what a service it was! What Howard said was so powerful, and the way the service was conducted made for such a joyous occasion. It was a great send-off for Mom. I am so happy to have that memory.

Howard also married my wife Darcy and me on his birthday! He baptized my son James and my daughter Dylan. He is indeed a great friend and someone I respect a great deal. As it comes with the territory of his calling, Howard is always on his way to the hospital or to be at the side of those in need of comfort. I knew it would be great to have him say a few words about how caregiving affects people and families and how important respite care is to care-givers.

## Reflections on being a Pastoral Caregiver by the Rev. L. Howard Maltby, St. Alban's Episcopal Church, Lexington, South Carolina.

My reflections are based on more than 25 years as an ordained Episcopal priest serving full-time for my whole ministry in congregations large and small. I have not been a "care-giver" of a loved one who is experiencing diminishing ability to care for him or herself. I am beginning to have more personal experience with this as my parents are in their 80s and my father is becoming more of a care-giver to my mother. Mostly, I am the "pastoral" care-giver to the care-giver as well as the one for whom they care. By "pastoral" care-giver, I mean that I am the one who supports others in their sacred journey through life. I represent God and the church to people. Therefore I try to present myself as compassionate and loving.

Because they "don't know what to say," it is common for people to step away from those who need care and attention. I was fortunate to receive an insight into effective pastoral care very early in my training. The expression which applies to my approach is I aim to be a "non-anxious presence." So often the one needing care primarily wants reassurance that they are not alone. Many times I simply sit by their bed, holding their hand, and let them rest, or let them talk about whatever is on their mind. They just want to feel loved. My focus now shifts to caring for the care-giver. The range of emotions and stages of grief and loss will vary from one person to another. (The whole range of those same emotions is found in one person over time). I draw from a basic tenet of St. Benedict's rule for monastic life. The importance of "balance" between worship, work, and recreation has contributed to the health and well-being of monastic communities for centuries. It is also beneficial to individual and family life. The stress of being a care-giver is difficult for the non-care-giver to fully comprehend.

One aspect not named in the stages is the guilt one has for experiencing anger at a loved one who is no longer the person they fell in love with, and with whom they shared life. Being a non-anxious presence with the care-giver is a useful practice in such circumstances. Depending on the personality of the care-giver, there may need to be some guidance offered on self-care. Good self-care includes maintaining the balance mentioned above. How that is accomplished calls for intentional planning. There are as many different ideas on how to carve out some "me time" as there are situations crying out for self-care options. From the briefest to longer, may I suggest; Respite care – every care giver needs a break! A few hours away from the loved one are beneficial to both. There is the obvious benefit of allowing the care-giver to attend to their own personal needs like having their hair done or taking in a movie, which offers a distraction to the mind and relieves one of worry for a short time. Additionally, having a different care-giver from time to time provides another set of eyes to observe subtle changes in the loved one, which may go unnoticed by the same person with them round the clock.

Adult day care has structured programs for your loved one and may be staffed by professionals offering needed activity and therapy. While your loved one is being looked after for an entire day, you have even greater opportunity to divert your attention to something you haven't been able to do, or see someone you haven't seen in too long. A retreat: This can be "Sabbath" time for rest and restoration. To avoid care-giver burn out, accumulating feelings of anger at things that one can't change, and guilt for feeling the way you do from time to time, a retreat could be a significant resource. There are numerous "retreat houses" around the country, operated by religious communities. One may arrange for a "guided" retreat with a member of the community offering time to meet and assist you with looking at your life situation. Or an "unguided" retreat allows one to immerse himself or herself in the ordered life of the community and engage at their level of comfort. A minimum of three days is suggested for the greatest benefit. One should expect that the first day will be spent disengaging from the world and the weight of it, which you are carrying on your shoulders. The second day should be full of rest and rejuvenation. The third day is when one begins the transition back to your world. It may be possible to find a retreat with a leader who has experience working with care-givers. In conclusion, I look at what I believe I am facing within my own family, as well as imagining how I would like to be cared for when my abilities diminish. The care-giver and the one being cared for share an unpleasant reality. That is loss of control over... too many things to mention. We struggle to attain some level of control in such situations.

As a pastoral care-giver, I try to assist people in finding the little things to highlight as evidence of still being in control. The "big picture" is beyond our ability to change, but we do control how we respond to it. Before I leave a pastoral care visit, I pray with those present. I hold up in my prayers the people involved, even when not present, the situation, health care providers, and I call on God to bless it all. I believe God can transcend our hang-ups and transform what looks sad to joy. The love of God in Jesus Christ redeemed humanity and the love of God in each of us can bring peace to even the most dire situation.

Bless you care-givers. Thank you for making significant sacrifices for those you love.

I wrote this book for you, the care-giver.
Maybe the next few pages about saying goodbye are for me.
You may decide if it is helpful or not for you at this time.

This Ice Cream is Delicious

# 12.

Mom's health began to rapidly decline and then, she fell. The nurse told me she was having some pain and we found out she had fractured her hip bone/pelvis. I ordered a wheelchair. Man, let me tell you, she looked way out of place in that chair. It didn't suit her at all. I was called in for a meeting with the staff, and I knew it was going to be about moving Mom to the nursing part of the Lowman Home. This was the last move.

On a Wednesday we moved her things into her new room. I took her for one more stroll around the pond where we ended a lot of our visits by feeding the fish and turtles. She was in her wheelchair, looking down. She was so confused, so weak, so frail, and so tired. We stopped and I parked her wheelchair in the warm sun. I sat down next to her, held her hand and asked my Creator for mercy and understanding.

I asked for an end.


Thursday we moved Mom into her new room. By then she wasn't talking at all. Occasionally she would nod but I wasn't sure if she understood anything. I was as sad as a son can be.

I received a call the following Saturday night from Nan, the head nurse and one of the most wonderful people I have ever met. Nan told me I needed to come back and be with Mom. So I made my last drive home to see Mom. I had been saying goodbye to her in small ways for the last eight years and now it had come to these final days. Words can't describe them. I'll just say I sat by her side with our family and her best friends. Six days later, on Friday, October 31, 2008, she died a completely natural death. No science. No tubes.

Exactly the way she wanted it.

The morning before I received that heartbreaking call from Nan, Ardis and Kay stopped by to see Mom. They brought her favorite food, ice cream.

She hadn't said a word in months so something I could only describe as a miracle happened. Mom took one bite and said:

"This ice cream is delicious."

# Acknowledgments

## Thank You

First and foremost I want to thank my wife Darcy for her support, understanding, patience and love. She knows more than anyone what I went through with Mom. I was gone the first three years of our marriage physically and mentally, but she knew my priority had to be Mom. I owe her some time along with our two small children James Sumter (4) as in "General Thomas Sumter – The Fighting Gamecock" and our daughter, Dylan Alexander (2) as in "Bob." Darcy had the kids a lot of weekend mornings for almost a year and a half so I could write this. I'm back now. The book is done! Hello Darcy, my beautiful wife!

I want to thank my dad. Life was dishing out some rather harsh times and he coached me through a lot of the rough spots. As I mentioned, he is the one who encouraged me to write this book. Thanks Dad, for all your love and support. You have always been "there" for me and through the years you have taught me what being a good father is all about. You are the best dad a son could ever have.

I was lucky, not only did I have two great parents but I am fortunate to have an incredible step mother. Martha had gone through AD with her father, so she knows. She was such a help with grammar, punctuation, and gave great suggestions about rephrasing ideas and statements. She is a terrific lady and has been such a blessing for my dad and me. Dad meeting Martha is just the best thing that could have happened to my family and her son, Walker, is my brother in every way.

I want to thank my aunts Mary Beth and Poochie. They are without a doubt the best sisters Mom could have and the best aunts I could ever have. Like I said earlier, I come from a very loving family and I consider that to be the greatest of all blessings. I'd also like to thank my uncles, Gary and Roger and all my cousins – Phil, Mac and Sandie, Melissa, Elizabeth, Jancy, Alice, Katie, Duncan, Jared, Hailey, Chad, Will, Maryann and Atti!

My mother-in-law Chris helped me organize my interviews and encouraged me the whole way. She understood my need to write and always had confidence in what I was doing. I am so thankful to her and my father-in-law Gary. Their house is such a wonderful home away from home for our family. The weekends Darcy and the kids spent there really allowed me the time I needed to write this book.

Thanking Mom's best friends Kay and Ardis is just not enough. They are truly the best friends anyone could have.

I would like to thank the families with whom I have worked. To be able to do what I do is a privilege. I appreciate you inviting me into your lives, allowing me to earn your trust and in return, trusting me to work with your loved one. To the spouses, daughters, and sons; I am in awe of your struggles. It's is unbelievably difficult to be a primary care-giver and I can't even begin to imagine what a lot of you are going or have gone through: Shelly, Anna and Sara, Beth, Jan, Gerri, Cornelia, Anne, Phil, Lisa, Pearl Ann, Larry and Elis, Scott, Tim, Lee, L.T., Tommy, Gene, Fletcher, Elaine and Teresa, E., Carol and Beth K., and Thomas. Scott was the first hombre with whom I worked and felt as though I was making a difference. The inspiration for "The Lodge" came from working with him. Both Shelly and I learned a lot together in those years. Through my work I have gotten to know a lot of great people and their families. I am thankful for that opportunity.

Wendy Klare. As I said earlier, writing a birthday card is agony for me so how this book happened is still a mystery. Actually, writing it was easy. I just sat down and wrote what was on my mind, as you probably could tell, but the editing, that was the difficult part. Without my friend Wendy and her guidance this book would have clocked in at over a thousand pages and would have been unreadable. It's not often you find someone with real talent who will help with almost no pay, take their time, and give it 100 percent. I appreciate all your help Wendy. I really can't thank you enough.

The Reverend Howard Maltby. My great friend Howard who presided over some of the most important events in my life. You are a representative of all the good things in this world. I'm so grateful you were here to see this book before you left us. When I hear 'Crown Him With Many Crowns' I will always think of you.

I'd like to thank a number of doctors and neurologists throughout Atlanta, in particular, Doctor Lah and Doctor Levey (Director, Emory Alzheimer's Disease Research Center). Their trust in my work has helped to make Let's Go a success. I appreciate their entire staff. I'd also like to thank Doctor

Charles M. Shissias, Neurology of the Low Country Medical Group, for his early guidance and perspective. And Martha Ehlenbeck for her nursing expertise.

I'd like to thank my interviewees. They took their time (nothing more important than time) to help me write this book. I have interviewed the best of the best and I hope their advice gives you some peace of mind. I'd like to thank Claire Reid, who knew that what I was doing was a little different and more involved than normal companionship. She was always encouraging me to be the best I can be and to make Let's Go something special. Her thumbs-up review of the rough draft for this book encouraged me beyond words. I'd like to say thanks to all my close pals whom I ignored for years but who always asked how Mom was doing: Jim, Chip, Britt, Stevie, Jack, Dan, Jeff G., Jeff C. Joey, John, David, Peter, Michael, Marcus, Lawrence, Kevin, Paul, Suzette, Perry, and James. I appreciate your friendship beyond words. My good friend, Mike Cuccarro for my contract. All the families agree – great contract! Josh, for his help with my first brochure. It had 5000 words on it and was unreadable, but his cartoon character logo was perfect! I'd like to thank Patrick Boggs – my friend and drummer pal for the Let's Go and The Lodge web sites and all things related to the wonderful world of computers of which I know very little. Pal, Jonny (One Take) Whiteside, for some of the graphics with earlier fliers. Gregory Nicoll for advice about interviewing and information about publishing... Gracias Amigos! The Reverend Beth Gustafson and the Reverend Cheryl Gosa. Their early guidance and introductions toward local churches led to my first clients. I'd also like to thank all the wonderful and truly caring people I met at these churches, in particular Chris Moore-Keish Assoc. Pastor at First Presbyterian Church, Atlanta. I was so happy to be out of the world of competitive care-giving and into the world of real caring and compassion. I'd like to thank Sharon Steele at Meals on Wheels/Senior Connections in DeKalb County. Ginnie Plunkett at Meals On Wheels/Fayette Senior Services Life Enrichment Center. Cobb County Senior Services/Meals On Wheels in Austell. Meagan Reed and Kimoya Hill for being the best activities combo in Atlanta and Sherry McAdams for her early guidance on adult day care.

I knew that the blessing of the Alzheimer's Association was going to be important for Let's Go to be successful. I met with Suzette Binford, (Family Support Services Director) and Mia Chester (Community Services Coordinator). I remember their kind words and genuine encouragement. A week later I received a call – a referral from the Alzheimer's Association!

I'd like to thank Jane Elliott and, of course, Kara Johnson. I appreciate everything you do.

Writing a book is a pretty lonely walk. It's exciting at times, but it's also easy to drive yourself crazy. Trying to finish this book (a process I was very unfamiliar with) was doing just that... driving me crazy. Anneke Smith's guidance in copy editing and her terrific suggestions/edits put me and the book on track at just about the time we were headed off the rails. Thanks Anneke – you have been a tremendous help. I'd like to thank my friend, Gwinn Bruns, for introducing me to Jane Shelton. Jane not only copy edited this book but she appreciated what I was saying and how I wanted to say it. From the first moment we talked, I knew instantly the book was in good hands. Thank you, Jane. You did an amazing job. I'd also like to thank my two proof-readers, Suzanne Carruthers, Mom of one of my best childhood pal's (Suzanne and I have been friends since I was six!) and my friend Kim Nielson, who is a modern day Super Woman, she proof-read this book with a two-week-old baby! Formatting, again another complicated process in this maze of finishing a book! When I met Rebecca Shaw I had a feeling that this was not only an important meeting, but meant to be. She formatted the book exactly the way I had envisioned it. She also helped me format a blueprint for getting these ideas to you. Thank you Rebecca, I am so glad to have met you. The ideas in any book are certainly crucial but not presenting them well is a waste of time. It's people like you all that make books worth writing and reading.

Special thanks to Frank Hunt for putting me to work as a young man and inspiring me to know that life is an adventure – one not to be missed.

Ellen Roberson. Having worked for her at Pace Travel I came to respect being an entrepreneur and knew one day I would start my own business. I'd like to thank all my friends, Donna, Trish, Doug and everyone at Pace Travel. I loved that job.

I'd like to thank John Lydon for teaching me that honesty is the code that all decent men live by.

...and last but not least I'd like to thank GiGi and Del. I appreciate your truly wonderful companionship and all the walks, trips to the river, warm welcomes home, and uncompromising, very real and beautiful friendship. You two made my life bearable when sometimes it seemed as though everything was falling apart. You are the most wonderful companions a man could ever have. You are my two best friends.

# Bibliography

**NOW**

1. Pg. 23 Paddock, Catharine, PhD, "Alzheimer's Amyloid Plaque Removal May Be Aided by Vitamin D and Omega 3", http://www. medicalnewstoday.com/articles/255957.php
2. Pg. 23 "Recommended Vitamins for Alzheimer's", http://www. livestrong.com/article/333537
3. Pg. 24 Alzheimer's Association, "Alternative mega-3 fatty acids", http:// www. alz.org/alzheimers_diseas_alternative_treatments.asp
4. Pg. 25 "Study: Exercise slows Alzheimer's brain atrophy, The Associated Press, Yahoo! News, July 27, 2008

**CONTROL**

1. Pg. 60 "Listen to the Music", Doobie Brothers, Toulouse Street, Warner, 1972
2. Pg. 60
"Isn't She Lovely", Stevie Wonder, Songs in the Key of Life, Motown, 1976
"I Walk the Line", Johnny Cash, Sun Records, 1955
"More than A Feeling", Tom Scholz/Boston, Boston, Epic Records, 1976
"Philadelphia Freedom", The Elton John Band, MCA, 1975
"Walkin' After Midnight", Patsy Cline, Decca, 1956
"Moonlight Serenade", Glenn Miller, RCA Bluebird, 1939
"Crusin", Smokey Robinson, Where There's Smoke..., Motown, 1979
"Heart of Glass", Blondie, Parallel Lines, Chrysalis, 1979

**A Progression of Care**

1. Pg. 132 "You Can't Always Get What You Want", Mick Jagger and Keith Richards, The Rolling Stones, Let It Bleed, London Records, 1969 Pg
2. Pg. 157 "Don't Worry, Be Happy", Bobby McFerrin, Simple Pleasures, 1988
3. Pg. 160 Brettell, Richard, PhD, "Museum Masterpieces: The Louvre", Course No. 7175, The Great Courses

**Appendix**

1. Pg. 209 "What's Going On", Marvin Gaye, Tamla Records, 1971

# Appendix

# The Question:

I have asked "the question" of several friends and colleagues who have experienced Alzheimer's with a loved one. I asked them to tell me what they would have done differently knowing what they know now. While these suggestions may not pertain to your particular situation they might inspire you to do something now before it's too late.

———————————

"I wish I had known something about dementia during the early stages of Paul's dementia. Instead of being able to control the circumstances surrounding the approach of dementia in a thoughtful, meaningful way, the dementia took over and controlled the entire course of events. Just as I would begin to understand what was going on with Paul, the dementia would take a new, unexpected, twist. The dementia was clearly in charge."

"I wish I would have been more patient in the beginning and asked Stan more questions about his memory. In my denial, I thought he was just being stubborn."

"From my own experience, a topic that is probably not so uncommon – the loved one who has been diagnosed or may need to be diagnosed with Alzheimer's, second to a disease they are already fighting. Because my Mom was in a struggle with Lymphoma, her AD symptoms were being ignored by her doctors, and consequently all of her children to some degree. We were asking questions about her short-term memory loss but getting no adequate response. Her family doctor just kept saying it was stress, exhaustion, perhaps a side effect of chemo. Imagine my shock when her primary cancer doctor at Duke said he would not treat her cancer any further (a tumor appeared in her lungs) because of her dementia. It was his policy not to treat a patient who had dementia. Up until this point no one would acknowledge the memory issues and then all of a sudden they were so significant that her life-saving cancer treatment would be denied? My advice for the care-giver, make sure you are seeing legitimate AD medical support when you suspect a problem just as if you had no other medical issues. Then, on a level playing field, you and all the doctors can sort out the best course. Be sure the AD doesn't get ignored. Perhaps things would have been no different for us but I would like to have had all the information and choices."

"Eating out. Great tip about finding a waitress and giving her a heads up about AD. Had I thought of this early on, I might not have been so reluctant to take Dad out."

"In the beginning, after my husband was diagnosed but still able to enjoy many things, I wish I would have made the effort and taken Phil to get certified in scuba diving. He has always wanted that and still talks about never doing it."

"I learned early on to completely avoid the use of the word "remember" when talking with Susan. No more "Do you, remember how much fun it was when we…" Instead I'll just say, "Susan, it is so much fun when we…"

"After Ed had to retire earlier than he wanted to because of his symptoms with AD, his friends rarely came by or called. I didn't really understand why until I realized that most of his friendships where through his business."

"Had I known just how confused she really was, a long time ago I would have simplified her clothing options to just a few of her favorites."

"When mentioning names of others in a conversation with Mom, I learned over time the importance of making this easier on her. For example, I'll say, "Mom, my husband George…" Or, "Mom, my oldest daughter and your first granddaughter Anne Collier…"

"I wish I would have taken Mom out to California to see her sister one last time before her dementia had really taken control. I thought about it for years but never got around to doing it."

"I would have moved Dad into assisted living before, or at least no later, than the day I had to unplug his stove. There were so many signs that he needed real help, an obvious one being the number of times I approached his apartment only to be alarmed by the smell of a burnt pan waffling in the hallway outside his door. Dangerous."

"Watching a true pickup in Mom's level of happiness, watching her appetite bounce back, and observing her total enjoyment in the assisted living facility (something I could have never imagined in her pre-dementia days) made it crystal clear that Mom was now where she needed to be."

"Again, along the same lines, I now know the huge benefit of a 100% memory care facility vs. the typical assisted living facility. No comparison. The fact that every single activity planned each day is for someone just like Mom is a huge plus. No longer is she in a place where much of the energy seems to go to the assisted living residents, while the memory care residents are placed in front of a TV, with occasional low-key activities planned for them."

Knowing what I know now, I wished we would have taken more trips together and gone out to eat more, but I didn't know how long she would live. No one knows that, so you have to pay attention to the bank account. Err on the side of reason and make rational choices. We saved our money, and we were lucky. Mom didn't have to live in a nursing home for six months or three years when that level of care is really expensive. I had always assumed that she would run out of money before the end of her life.

"I'd like to say to all the care-givers, to get through this, you are going to need all the help you can get: through relatives, friends, clergy, work friends, support groups, and temporary care-givers. It's there. Sometimes you have to look for it. Sometimes you have to ask for it but most importantly, you need to realize, help rarely comes on its own."

# 50 Things

## What you can do right now:

1. Daily planner: Write out things on a **paper** calendar. If YLO used a daily planner in his or her life before AD, you are in good shape. Let them get used to reading it every morning and periodically checking back. If they never used one before, now is a good time to start. Write out things that need to get done: chores, yard work, appointments. Challenge them a bit.

2. Set up a Facebook or Caring Bridge account. Caring Bridge also has a feature for organizing tasks and coordinating care. This might be a great way for a grandchild or niece/nephew to help out. They both are great ways to let everyone know what is going on in YLO's life. Keep everyone in the loop.

3. Take that trip if finances allow. If you think she might still enjoy a trip to Spain... go! Go sailing. Do whatever that "big deal" was he or she was always talking about. Use the time you have together to the fullest.

4. Cell phones: While visiting someone with AD, lower the ringer. When you accept or make a call, step away. Most people with AD are "living in the now." Cell phones can be very distracting and "exclusive."

5. Have a few business cards or small notes that state the person with you has Alzheimer's, and all questions should be directed to you. Great for restaurants.

### Realize:

6. The hard part about AD is not taking everything personally. Don't forget that it's the disease, not them and not you!

7. Believe in what you are doing. If you think a certain medication or regimen is working, then it is working. You know YLO the best. You can recognize the small changes better than anyone else.

8. AD is hard to understand because the symptoms can vary with each person. I have worked with people where there are gradual changes over time, but I have worked with others where I notice changes with almost every visit. Sometimes there is just no explanation why someone just stops eating their favorite foods, refuses to leave the house, or becomes so reliant on their spouse they just <u>have</u> to be in the same room with them.

Most care-givers are constantly seeking answers and trying to understand the changing behavior of their loved one. Sometimes you can find a reason and a solution for a certain behavior; sometimes you can't. At a certain point I believe when there are no crystal clear answers, looking for a reason for a certain behavior can be far more stressful than just accepting the changes in YLO.

9. A client's wife once jokingly asked me when she forgot something, "Is dementia contagious?" I told her "Not biologically, but the confusion is!"

10. We all have our good and bad days and those with AD/dementia are no different.

11. Every family is different. Every person is different. I take my clients out in public as long as I know I have enough control, and I also know that there is a strong possibility they will enjoy the outing. I took my Mom out to restaurants, the movies and to see her friends up until the very end. I think that was appropriate and I know in my heart she appreciated the effort. But, I have also taken people to social gatherings and events that they did not enjoy.

Taking people out of their homes and getting them out in the world is what I do. My goal is to try and restore self-esteem and pride. When it comes to making decisions about YLO attending ceremonies, church, parties, and events, only you can make decisions like these. I would recommend to always consider what YLO **would have wanted** as well what they may want now.

**Important revisits:**

**Chapter 1  Now**

12. Proper nutrition: "An apple a day."

13. Daily exercise: Get the legs moving and the blood flowing. Exercise builds appetite and promotes good sleep. Start walking every day. Look for a place close by where you two can walk indoors when the weather is bad.

14. Going back to work: I will assume that YLO is no longer employed, so finding worthwhile activities to do is important. Volunteering.

## Chapter 2  Control

15. Safety First: #1 Safety. #2 Budget. #3 Happiness. Safety is your number one responsibility as a care-giver. Happiness is something to strive for. Since YLO's safety is your number one concern take a few precautionary steps to make YLO's home a safe environment. (visit Alz.org, look under Caregiver Center/Home Safety).

16. Routines, Repetition, Rituals and Habits: Routine will allow someone with AD to stay more focused. It adds structure to their day and gives everyone more control.

17. Simplifying, Downsizing and De-cluttering: Clutter just adds to confusion. See the interview with "Martha Stewart."

18. Going places and leaving the house: Realize that getting ready to go somewhere might take a little longer. Build in more time to that part of the day.

19. Locks and keys: Change all house locks to one uniform lock. Part of the "simplify plan."

20. Your tone of voice: Conversations between you should not sound any different than ten years ago on your end. Always, always respect their mind. Do not talk to YLO as though he or she is a child.

21. When I'm a bit stressed, my kids pick up on it immediately. It transfers. It's no different with someone who has AD. Your calm demeanor will help reduce YLO's level of anxiety.

22. Asking YLO "Why are you doing this?" or "Why are you acting this way?" will probably not get you the explanation you were looking for. Sometimes they don't know why.

23. I give my clients control by allowing them to make as many choices as possible. If they think they have a choice that makes for a much more enjoyable experience for everyone.

24. In turn, as AD progresses, too many choices for YLO can be too confusing. Make it easier. Example: Instead of saying "Would you like spaghetti or Chinese food for dinner?" say, "Would you like spaghetti for dinner?"

25. Buy DVDs and CDs of favorite programs and music: They will give you time to catch up on your life when YLO is watching and listening. Favorite movies, *Ellen,* or *Gunsmoke.* It all works.

26. Evaluate driving: Should they still be driving? Are they dangerous to themselves and more importantly… to others?

27. The dentist: I took a client to a dentist that specialized in people who have dementia. He was kind, considerate, and patient. Check in your area for one if you have had a difficult time getting YLO to see a dentist.

28. Replacing: Introducing new TV remote controls, gadgets, and other equipment is not a good idea. If what you have works, keep it.

**Chapter 3  Rx**

29. Depression: If you had just been told you have Alzheimer's, wouldn't you be depressed? Look into antidepressants or anti-anxiety medications.

30. Getting the right combination of medicines to work can take some time. It can be an ongoing process, so have some patience with YLO's doctor who is trying to prescribe the right balance of helpful meds.

31. It's crucial to monitor and manage medications. Don't allow YLO to suffer from possible side effects from these medications when there are other medication options.

**Chapter 4  Family Business**

32. See an elder law attorney/financial advisor: Plan for the future. You need to know your care options, what you can afford, and the laws in your state regarding long-term care, Medicare, and Durable Power of Attorney. It's also time to create a real budget where a financial advisor has consulted with your family. Stick to it. Smart money management is vital when the future is uncertain. Get to know how Medicare works and what you will be responsible for.

33. Set up a family plan of action: As a family and as care-givers, it's your responsibility to work together. Realize that getting along with your siblings while caring for your parents is the best compliment you can give them.

**Chapter 5  Information**

34. Classes at the Alzheimer's Association: If you don't have a local branch take them on-line.

35. Look into attending an Alzheimer's support group: They aren't for everyone but they might be for you.

36. Safe Return: An identification jewelry program that assists in the safe return of individuals with dementia who wander and become lost.

## Chapter 6   Sandra, Rosebud, Poochie, and Mary Beth

37. A personal history: Start collecting important letters, documents, and pictures for a folder YLO can look at from time to time. This will help them remember who they are and give visitors some ideas about topics of conversation. Start collecting favorite photographs and letters for "Your Book."

## Chapter 10   A Progression of Care

38. When considering assisted living for YLO, look back ten years ago when they were of sound mind and body. Was there a plan? Would they have said, "I do not want to be a burden to you?" Keep with the original plan. It's what YLO wanted.

39. Contact: Some of my clients are just forgetful. They can still focus, still enjoy activities and getting out is fun. Sometimes they are maybe even eager to experience something new. On the other hand I have clients who (mostly in the later stages) are not only forgetful but their minds are constantly at work, almost racing. I can start a conversation but in a matter of seconds they have already moved on. Their minds seem to be headed towards the future or the past or a confusing mixture of both so talking about the present, what is happening right now, can be difficult. When considering a move into assisted living I think being surrounded by things that are familiar; pictures, furniture, music, TV shows, movies, and books are not only comforting but being surrounded by these might give you a better chance at making "contact."

40. Assisted Living: $3,000.00 or more, a month, times how many years YLO might be staying there, adds up to lot of money so you should expect nothing less than what they said they would deliver. Start a network with the other residents' families and friends so you can share information and observations. (Swap email addresses and phone numbers). Work "together" in making sure the level of care your loved ones are receiving is appropriate. The more people looking out for YLO the better off he/she will be. **As consumers we have the power to make a difference.**

41. A helpful staff makes all the difference: If you can't get the attention of anyone or you can't make eye contact at the nursing station, that generally is an indication they are inattentive. Let a manager know your concerns.

42. Posted on the wall, usually by the elevator is a sign that says "Ombudsman." That is your "go to" government agency in case you see any abuse.

43. When things start to get misplaced and especially when you are thinking about moving YLO into assisted living, consider going to a jeweler for ring fittings. Some day he might lose his wedding ring because it's too loose. Get it refitted smaller for a tighter fit.

44. Diamonds and jewelry: Before you move YLO into assisted living or hire a care-giver, you might want to consider replacing the diamond in her ring with a glass replica. Jewelry stores offer this service.

## Chapter 11  Overwhelmed

45. Respite Care – care for the care-giver. You need to take care of yourself so you can be the best care-giver you can be. That means taking time for you and taking a break from Alzheimer's.

46. Stress: Your level of stress is through the roof so slow down. That stress will exploit the weakness in your own body and might lead to all kinds of physical problems. That means you need to take care of your body. You are going to need your health.

47. Going on a trip with friends and getting away from your responsibilities for a few days will help make you a better care-giver. Go to the party you were invited to. Go out to dinner with friends. Do not feel guilty. You have earned it and YLO wants you to go!

48. Telling close friends about YLO's Alzheimer's diagnosis can bring a sense of relief from hiding it and being in denial.

49. When you see changes in YLO, tell friends about those changes, especially if they are ever alone with YLO, so they don't think that the behavior is a reaction toward them.

50. Always remember: Your loved one who has Alzheimer's wants the best for you. The last thing in the world they would want is for you to worry yourselves sick. What your loved one wants, more than anything, is for you to be happy.

This is a survey that I give to the care-givers of potential new clients. It might help you organize your thoughts.

**SURVEY**

Let's GO
CAREGIVERS' ASSISTANCE

Date _____

**If you would like to meet, please have the survey completed. Help me get to know your loved one and be better prepared to help you.**

**Primary Caregiver:**

Name: _____Relationship: _____

Contact Information (Phone, email): _____

**Your Loved One:**

Name: _____ Age: _____

Lives Where (Neighborhood): _____

Born Where: _____

Grew Up Where: _____

Education: _____

Military Service: _____

Occupation/Profession: _____

Hobbies/Interests: _____

_____

Organizations / Charities /Religious Affiliation: _____

_____

Siblings: _____

Friends: _____

Current Level of Activity: _____

Diagnosed When/ By Whom: _____

How is your loved one coping with the diagnosis?

Sad___ Angry___ Depressed___ Indifferent___ Anxious___ In denial___

Other: _____

How are you coping with the diagnosis? _____

Have you seen an Elder Law attorney? Y__ N__

Do you have Power of Attorney? Y__ N___

Is there a will? Y__ N___ Living Will? Y__ N___

Have any antidepressant/anti-anxiety medications been prescribed?
Y__ N___

What side effects are there? _____

Have any anti-delusional medications been prescribed?

Are there side effects? _____

Are you participating in an Alzheimer's support group? Y__ N___

Are other family members involved at this stage? Y__ N___

If yes, list names: _____

Are you comfortable with the level of support you are receiving from family and friends? Y__ N___

What else should we know? Please fill in any other information about the situation:

_____

_____

_____

_____

_____

_____

Let's GO
CAREGIVERS' ASSISTANCE
www.AtlantaLetsGo.com

# An Interview with Liam

I met Liam at a support group lunch sponsored by the Alzheimer's Association. He introduced himself, said some kind words about this book and as we continued I felt like I could have talked to him for a week! I found this conversation to be profound on two different levels. One, it was the first in-depth conversation I had about the book with a total stranger and second and more importantly, Liam has Alzheimer's. He was diagnosed a year ago. (I have to say that Liam's reading and comprehension ability's are exceptional for someone diagnosed with AD.)

Hello Liam,

It's been terrific getting to know you. I hope this interview will offer some perspective to families and healthcare professionals.

**Q. What does a family usually overlook in regards to how to talk about Alzheimer's with someone with AD?**

A. *Don't think about us having Alzheimer's. Talk to us as if we were (and we are!) the same person. Our symptoms when you meet us after our diagnosis are probably not visible. We don't initially have problems-mobility problems, stuttering, inability to choose the correct word, a dazed look that are visible. Just talk your normal way, complete with humor, sarcasm, etc.*

**Q. What worries you the most about being diagnosed with AD?**

A. *That's easy. Some people with AD know about the disease, its progression but not its speed, and the eventual conclusion. It's natural to think about the progression and if it is happening before our eyes. NOT thinking about it is hard to do. Filling your day with exercise, reading, socializing, using your brain minimizes your worrying and you can see you are NOT deteriorating.*

**Q. Why do you think there isn't a better system of care for people who have dementia?**

A. *Slow, inaccurate evaluation by medical professionals and their tests; slow, weak information from dementia-related groups – probably nationwide; weak and/or inconsistent information and publicity from media, nonprofit organizations, corporations.*

**Q. What could our communities do better as far as offering services for families?**

A. *A difficult question. The solution is based on fiscal investment by all levels of government that needs to continue for a long time. "Better" will require changes in allocation of funds. I know that some countries have faced problems differently and with success.*

**Q. What is one thing about having AD that people might not be able to comprehend?**

A. *We are still compassionate, thinking individuals regardless of our difficulties.*

**Q. For the primary care-giver, support and understanding from friends and family is very important. What do you think is the main reason that a family member or friend can't accept a diagnosis, won't participate or offer help?**

A. *Main reason – Ignorance/weak-poor understanding/knowledge of AD being a brain disease. Our friends are in our age bracket. They have memory problems and think OUR memory problems are similar to THEIR memory problems which they are NOT. These family and friends would have a better understanding of us if there were a way to have us live with them for a few weeks.*

# "What's Going On?"[1]

## Alzheimer's is Different

The numbers are staggering. One in eight older adults has dementia; soon, it will be one in seven. Alzheimer's is not like cancer. You can't have surgery for it and then get better. AD is a steady financial drain. People can live many years with it, and toward the end, help is usually needed. Alzheimer's is one of the scariest diseases out there; the one that really is the great illness of our generation. There are a lot of different organizations and senior centers that offer exceptional services for the care-giver, but I have to say, there doesn't appear to be cohesiveness or connection between them. Along with it being difficult to find out what our communities have to offer, it has been very difficult for me to find specific activities offered by anyone, any group or organization for those with dementia. I think this is the main reason we all feel like we are alone in this. It's because we are.

Based on my experience I have a few ideas and inexpensive suggestions...

### The County

- A Community Garden: The county could donate a plot of unused vacant land and split it up into individual plots for gardens with pathways. Put up fencing to keep the rabbits out. I love to garden. So did Mom. Watch the tomatoes and cucumbers grow.

- The County Rec center (the one that is empty all day until the kids get out of school). Twice a month, open the doors for people with dementia. Volunteers could be there to take YLO off your hands for an hour. A walk around the track. Maybe a few games. Basketball. Ping Pong. Light exercise. The care-giver could mingle with other care-givers, swap stories – a casual support group.

- The county could sponsor a day out in the spring and fall, such as a walk-a-thon event. "Save the river." Run by volunteers and at a high school track. Invite all to walk to raise money and awareness for something. It would be discreet and disguised so your loved one does not feel stigmatized.

- Volunteering: Volunteer programs should be established across the nation for those with early memory loss. It doesn't make sense to have so many people forced into early retirement who are still capable, willing and excited to go to work. It's all part of the unimaginative and static health care system we have. No one is thinking this through.

  **SOLUTION**: The AARP and the AMAC could organize the program – both are tied into many senior organizations and businesses.

  **Examples**: After school tutors. My 5 year old son's after school program is 400 kids in a cafeteria. People with early dementia who love kids could help with homework, drawing and activities from 3:00 to 5:00 every day. Bus monitors for elementary school – help out the driver by keeping things calm. Others: Meals on Wheels, food banks, professional visitors for those in assisted living.

  What you can do. Call the AARP (1-888-OUR-AARP) and AMAC (1-888-262-2006) OR send an email at to AARP.org under "Contact Us" send a message like: "My _____ has early memory loss and we are looking to volunteer. Do you have a program set up in our community?" Use this opening to find out what is going on in your area.

  AARP describes themselves as: "...a nonprofit, nonpartisan organization, with a membership of more than 37 million, that helps people turn their goals and dreams into real possibilities, strengthens communities and fights for the issues that matter most to families..."

  Seems to me this is a great place to start.

- Driving Assessment: You have become worried about your parent or spouse driving: A two hour written and driving test at the DMV for a scary teen-ager is about $20.00. In two area hospitals in Atlanta a "Driving Evaluation" for 60 year old who is diagnosed with dementia is $1,000.00. I guess if Mario Andretti or Burt Reynolds is doing the assessment then that would be OK, but a $1,000.00 seems a little high. I'm sure the price discourages a few families who really need the guidance.

SOLUTION: Our local county or state government should handle this by offering a "senior driving assessment." Let's take the profit out of a driving evaluation while making an effort to keep our roads safe for all drivers.

## Hospitals

- A Psychiatric Evaluation in Limbo.

There needs to be a place where a family can go to develop a care plan, for instance, for someone who has become delusional and aggressive. During this challenging time primary care-givers miss work, kids miss school, neighbors are confused, it's chaos in the house and **it's dangerous.**

There should be a better system in place that can direct families towards the resources they need. The current system, where you would take YLO to a psychiatric hospital for an evaluation is certainly important but advice about the next step can be vague. It's limbo at its finest and sometimes you have to figure out what to do by trial and error. Some families have a hellish, all-consuming problem on their hands even when they move their loved one into an assisted living "We finally found the right facility for Dad but will they kick him out if...?" This question is on every one's mind. But if it happens so often, (and it does) why is there such secrecy about what to do?

The system we have is ridiculously inadequate for this reason: Most state hospitals disappeared in the 80's. They were replaced by "magic medication" and an explosion of "for profit" assisted living facilities – FINE – but someone forgot to take into consideration that sometimes these miracle-anti-delusional drugs don't work. This 'someone' also forgot to open a few facilities that can manage these more complicated situations for a reasonable price.

Sorry, $10,000.00/month is not reasonable. That is a short path to bankruptcy. We all know it, but no one will do anything about it because there are too many people, making too much money, with too much influence.

This is a huge problem with no simple or quick solution. I am just raising the issue.

## Assisted Living Communities

- I think placing someone into assisted living is hard because there are so few standards among the facilities. Every facility has its own rules! Example: Community Fee. A community fee or move-in fee is between $1,000 and $3,000 and is usually non-refundable. After you hand over a community fee of $2,000.00 what happens if YLO is asked to move after two months? Since there is no standard practice it's up to the facility to either return the money (or not) or maybe give a partial refund. Of course in my experience most of the time guess who keeps the money? Yep. It's a very expensive cycle for some families.

**SOLUTION**: Ask the question before filling out an application *"If my husband is asked to leave because of behavioral problems will you refund my community fee?"* If they say *"No"* then keep looking and tell them this policy is unacceptable. This action will help change this bad and abusive policy. There should be a guaranteed full refund up to six months and partial refund up to one year. This should be adopted by every assisted facility licensed by any state in the United States. Make this a non-issue. The problem is lack of standards... this will help. Again, give the AARP and AMAC a ring.

If enough families ask this question **change would come immediately!**

To me, it's a little strange to try and lock a family down with a non-refundable fee when the world knows, or should know, how unpredictable dementia is. With the transition to memory care, in two instances, by the time the paperwork was signed my client's health had deteriorated so much that they needed to be in nursing care.

Some families need the freedom to choose the best place they can afford and not be trapped by this fee.

Let's make it a refundable deposit.

**The State**

- Why is it so difficult to get an ID for someone who has AD?

Here is an email that I received from Beth, Tom's wife:

> My husband started showing signs of dementia about ten years ago.
> A diagnosis of Alzheimer's disease came a few years later. Along
> with that diagnosis was the neurologist's order for my husband to
> stop driving. There was a very tumultuous period for us for at least
> a year. Even now, after three years, the subject comes up regularly
> about him wanting to drive.
>
> About a month ago, my husband misplaced/hid his wallet
> somewhere in our house. I believe it was to keep from having his
> license taken away. I thought this was a great opportunity for us to
> get a photo ID for him; issued by Georgia, but stating he could not
> drive. I went to the DMV (Department of Motor Vehicles) to request
> an application for the ID. The clerk told me that they would not issue
> an ID without the consent of the driver. I explained that my husband
> had AD and would never consent to relinquish his driver's license
> on his own. I offered to bring in the letter from his doctor saying
> that he was no longer allowed to drive. I also told her that since the
> new ID would look so much like a driver's license, it would satisfy
> my husband. She once again told me that they are "not allowed" to
> issue the ID without the permission of the driver.
>
> Trying to explain a rule or limitation to a person with AD is difficult.
> Getting them to give up something they've had all their adult lives
> is even harder. A little assistance from the DMV on this issue could
> make a world of difference in the stress level experienced by both
> the patient and the care-giver.

**Our Communities**

- Maybe we could convince the Humane Society to wave the three-hour
  orientation class for a few people who just want to participate in the
  dog walking. Drop that rule for a few people who will be supervised,
  and just let us walk a dog every now and then. There is no need for
  someone to have to sit through a three-hour orientation if they don't
  need to know how to run a cash register for the gift shop. All other
  programs, food banks, etc., take notice.

- Stressful Doctor Visits: The scheduling staff should pay attention to the time when they know a patient has dementia. Some people with AD can get restless and nervous, especially in a doctor's or dentist's waiting room, so be sure to tell the doctor and the staff that you are scheduling an appointment for a person who has AD and it is important to stick to the agreed time of the appointment.

## Organizations

### The Day Your Loved One is Diagnosed, What Do You Do?

- New care-givers don't have a clue about what to do or where to go and here is one reason why: From a neurologist's diagnosis to finding the right help can be a complicated maze. In Atlanta there are a thousand different organizations and businesses that address senior issues. That might be a good thing but it has been my experience that most of these organizations and businesses act like they don't know the others even exist. The world of dementia is a fractured one.

I believe that once a diagnosis has been made it would be advantageous if families in search of help and information were given all options – up front, completely void of competing interests. This is too important an issue to become a victim of cliques. It would be beneficial for healthcare providers, senior groups, senior centers and our communities to **work together**.

Information is vital for new care-givers, so I believe this cooperation would create a real path for families. That in itself would ease the burden of being a new care-giver. Finding help, looking for options for activities and support should be introduced as early as possible so families know what is available in the community and are not constantly wondering "What if" or "Is there something else out there?" Given all options for care and help – up front – will reassure families that they are doing everything possible for their loved one.

**Simply**: Alzheimer's is a condition that has unified a certain population and since it is now recognized as a disease instead of eccentricities there should be a better process of finding help in our communities.

- Sponsor a walking group. There is nothing better than walking – a one hour walk, twice a week outside, in a local gym or track can be very beneficial. A walking program can offer structure to families and AD patients. It's a smart way to battle the disease. Ask your local Alzheimer's Association (ALZ.org) to start a walking group. In Atlanta our local association partnered with the YMCA (YMCA.org) and we walk on a track, inside, twice a week, rain or 100 degrees. And it's FREE!.

- Local service organizations such as Rotary Club could sponsor indoor programs choosing simple to follow topics. For example, a talk about new light bulb technology and energy related issues. Not too complicated, yet informative enough that people feel engaged.

### Movies, Music and Art

- Movie Theaters: It would be great if one, *just one,* local movie theater played a classic, not too violent, movie during the day (say, at noon). Once a week on a weekday for people who want to see a movie but might think contemporary movies are just too much.

- Live Music: How about one bar or music venue having some live music for lunch? The only music I can find is usually classical music over at the local college or university. Most of my guys don't want to sit through an hour of 'avant garde' piano. Some churches do have music programs around lunchtime but I'm thinking a little more... fun. How about this: At a bar that is usually open during the day, patrons pay five bucks and get to listen to jazz/R&B or Rock-n-Roll while eating lunch. Pass out flyers to assisted living communities and you will have a packed house.

- Theater: I'm working with a guy now who used to be an actor down at the local community playhouse. I'm sure he would enjoy seeing a play. I bet a lot of people would love to see a play in the middle of the day. Every season an actor group could put on a play at one centrally located playhouse – a dress rehearsal open to the public. If it were advertised to the churches, synagogues, and retirement communities in the area, I bet the world would show up! There must be 250,000 retired folks living in Atlanta who would love to see a play in the middle of the day four times a year. Pay $7.00 and see a condensed one-hour play. Or how about a high school? Have Senior Day, where the production is put on for the "Real Seniors!" Open to the public, they could charge a few bucks and raise some money for the Theater Club. Everyone wins.

## Sports

- Golf camp: Is there a golf pro/instructor out there whose father has AD? You would know what these families are going through. How about organizing a camp for people who used to play golf but might have lost a step and some of their swing? It could be held twice a month in the spring and fall for two low peak hours, limited to four people, and each person pays $30. After the one-hour lesson, have a hot dog at the clubhouse while watching highlights of golf. The pro works two hours and makes $120.00 and helps four families. Challenging, fun, lunch, respite care... it's all there. The same goes for tennis.

- Fishing: There is almost no calmer activity. A fishing supply store could sponsor a "Community Support Program," and have a few mornings set aside for a "fishing rodeo."

- What if a local ball team donates to the Alzheimer's Association one parking space for a minivan/small bus and ten seats, four times a season for a day game. Same seats every time, in the shade. The parking space would be close to the seats so they are not too difficult to get to. Again, it's all here: Fun, socialization, lunch, and respite care.

- Local gymnasiums: A place with an indoor track that charges a minimal rate per hour to use only one part of the facility. For example, a gym has an indoor track that Christopher would love to use when it's raining or 110 degrees outside. He doesn't want to use the steam room or lift weights, just walk around the track for a half hour. Instead of paying the full $120.00/month rate how about $40? That would work great for the sponsored walking group.

- How about a volleyball league for those with early memory loss? Four on four. Make it fun and somewhat competitive, with team shirts, brackets, and pizza after. Don't call it anything special. Be very discreet. The players don't have to know its set up to accommodate people who have early AD. I bet there are at least sixteen people in Atlanta who have AD that would love to play volleyball. I work with two of them right now!

I think we need to at least give a few people who have Alzheimer's the opportunity to participate in something. I realize some people with dementia would never want to play volleyball, go for a hike, or walk through a museum. Sometimes just leaving the house is too much, so I know it's difficult to offer activities for many reasons: the stigmas attached, low self-esteem, depression, confusion and withdrawal. Even though it appears they can participate in these activities, it's difficult without supervision. The stages, personalities, and how it affects everyone are so different. Some people admit they have a problem and some won't admit to anything. How are we supposed to treat someone who can't do the things they used to do but at the same time, not tell them what to do in a group setting? It's hard. I think it's the main problem and why I have found it very difficult to find anything in Atlanta specifically designed for those who have mild to moderate AD. Most of the programs in day care or assisted living are geared toward the moderate to late stages where the activity is so simple or rudimentary that it often seems to some, *insulting.*

Alzheimer's is number one on most everyone's fear list, and as a culture, we seem to be paralyzed by that fear. *"Is this going to be how I end up?"* We pride ourselves on the amount of control we have over our lives. When we lose that control and become dependent on others, it's devastating in so many ways. However, with the lack of activities and options offered to people with AD, you would think Alzheimer's was an obscure disease, but it's not. It seems that everyone I talk to has been affected by it in some way.

I live in a city of five million people. Outside of adult day care and assisted living, it's hard for me to find any activities offered by anyone.

... SERIOUSLY?

AD is scary. I'm scared of it. My mom had it and her sister has it. It runs in my family, but you know what? If I get it, I hope I get to play volleyball. (Well, at least I hope I have the opportunity to play it if I want to.)

As a nation, it's time we bring Alzheimer's out of the closet and start talking about ways to help these families who are overwhelmed. We need to be discreet when it's called for, use specific strategies designed for all the different stages of Alzheimer's, and as a community find ways to improve the lives of our loved ones.

It's possible. I know it is.

Henry lives in Atlanta and is married with two children. Along with **Let's Go**, he manages a walking group with the Georgia Chapter of the Alzheimer's Association and is always on the look out for interesting and unique actives for his clients and those with Alzheimer's.

Made in the USA
Columbia, SC
07 October 2017